Nail Disorders

Common Presenting Signs, Differential Diagnosis and Treatment

Nail Disorders
Common Presenting Signs, Differential Diagnosis and Treatment

Robert Baran
MD

Head of Dermatology Department, General Hospital,
Cannes, France

Julian Barth
MB BS, MRCP

Senior Registrar in Dermatology, Department of
Dermatology, The Slade Hospital, Oxford, UK

Rodney Dawber
MA, MB, ChB, FRCP

Consultant Dermatologist, Department of
Dermatology, The Slade Hospital, Oxford, UK

CHURCHILL LIVINGSTONE
New York, Edinburgh, London, Melbourne, Tokyo

MARTIN DUNITZ

© **R Baran, JH Barth and RPR Dawber 1991**

First published in the United States in 1991
by Churchill Livingstone Inc, 1560 Broadway, New York, NY 10036

First published in the United Kingdom in 1991
by Martin Dunitz Ltd, 7–9 Pratt Street, London NW1 0AE

A catalog card for this book is available from the Library of Congress

ISBN 0-443-08800-4

Phototypeset by Scribe Design, Gillingham, Kent
Originated in Hong Kong by Imago Publishing Ltd
Printed and bound in Singapore by Imago Publishing Ltd

Contents

Preface

Most books in clinical medicine are written and organized according to disease classification—even though diseases present as symptoms and signs. For this reason, and also because nail apparatus signs are vividly obvious, we thought that a manual which took signs and outlined differential diagnoses might be useful to many doctors and paramedics involved with hand and foot diseases. The book is particularly aimed at those who are not trained in the details of many of the subtleties of more general skin or systemic diseases which might present with nail apparatus abnormalities. This type of book obviously requires colour illustrations and we sincerely hope that those selected are sufficiently clear and diverse to aid diagnosis.

This is not a book detailing diseases. If the reader requires more information we would recommend the following reference books:

Baran R and Dawber RPD, *Diseases of the nails and their management* (Blackwell Scientific Publications, Oxford 1984).

Samman PD and Fenton DA, *The nails in disease* (Heinemann, London 1986).

Zaias N, *The nail in health and disease* (Spectrum Publications, Jamaica, New York 1980).

RB
JHB
RPRD

Introduction

Without a normal nail unit on the most distal part of its dorsal surface, the many functions of any digit will be severely compromised. The nail apparatus adds subtle dexterity, protection and aesthetic adornment, particularly on the hands; the latter, 'cosmetic', function is as important as the others.

If one is to understand fully the pathogenesis of diseases affecting the nails then a detailed knowledge of the three-dimensional anatomy and physiology is mandatory — more so in this site than almost any other part of the integument, particularly if surgery is to be undertaken.

Therefore, before a description of the various symptoms and signs of disease in the sections that follow, it was considered appropriate to include diagrams outlining the basic structural components of the nail apparatus (see further Baran and Dawber, *Diseases of the nails and their management*, Ch 1) .

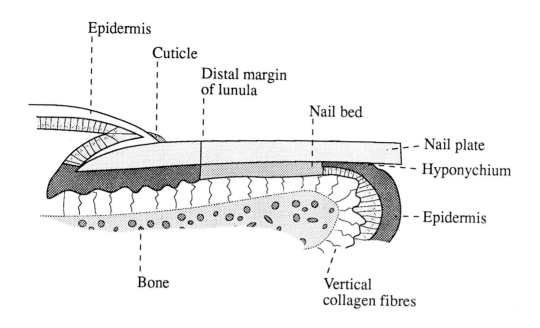

Epidermis
Cuticle
Distal margin of lunula
Nail bed
Nail plate
Hyponychium
Epidermis
Bone
Vertical collagen fibres

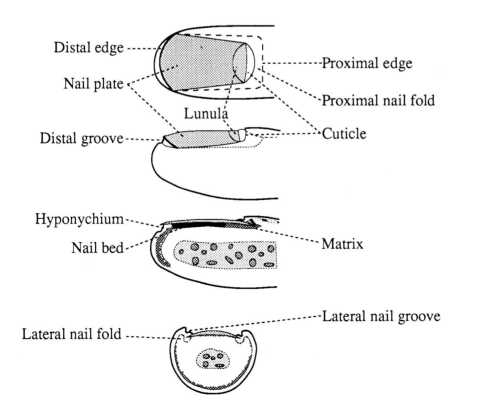

Distal edge
Proximal edge
Nail plate
Proximal nail fold
Lunula
Distal groove
Cuticle
Hyponychium
Nail bed
Matrix
Lateral nail groove
Lateral nail fold

1

Nail configuration abnormalities

Clubbing (Hippocratic fingers) (Figures 1.1–1.7)

The bulbous fingers showing the sign known as clubbing were described as long ago as the fifth century BC when Hippocrates noted such changes in patients suffering from empyema.

The morphological changes combine:
a) Bilateral curvature of the nails.
b) Enlargement of the soft tissue structures confined to the tips of the digits.

The increased nail curvature usually affects all twenty digits but may be particularly obvious on the thumbs, index and middle fingers.

The shape of the curved nails is variable and may appear fusiform, shaped like a bird's beak, or clubbed somewhat like a watch-glass.

There are four main categories of clubbing:

The simple type (Figures 1.1–1.4)

This is the most common category. It has several components:
a) Increased nail curvature with a transverse furrow which separates it from the rest of the nail both in the early stage and on resolution. The onset is usually gradual and painless, except in some cases of carcinoma of the lung where clubbing may develop abruptly and may be associated with severe pain.

b) Hypertrophy of the soft parts of the terminal segment due to a firm, elastic, oedematous infiltration of the pulp, which may spread on to the dorsal surface forming a periungual swelling.
c) Hyperplasia of the dermal fibro-vascular tissue which readily extends to involve the adjacent matrix. This accounts for one of the earliest signs of clubbing—that is, an abnormal mobility of the nail base which can be rocked back and forth giving the impression that it is floating on a soft oedematous pad. The increased vascularity is responsible for the slow return of colour when the nail is pressed and released.
d) Local cyanosis is present in up to 60 per cent of cases.

In the early stages clubbing may involve one hand only, though eventually both hands become affected symmetrically. Several stages of clubbing or acropachy may be distinguished: suspected, slight, average and severe. In practice the degree of the deformity may be determined by Lovibond's 'profile sign' which measures the angle between the curved nail plate and the proximal nail fold when the finger is viewed from the radial aspect. This is normally 160° but exceeds 180° in clubbing. With a modified profile sign one measures the angle between the middle and the terminal phalanx at the interphalangeal joint. In normal fingers the distal phalanx forms an almost straight (180°) extension of the middle phalanx, whereas in severe clubbing this angle may be reduced to 160° or even 140°. However, the best indicator may well be the measurement of the hyponychial angle. This may be assessed either clinically or with the aid of a clubbing 'shadow-graph' which may allow serial measurements of the angles to record any progression of the process. In fact, fixing the limits of true clubbing in minimal cases is ultimately a matter of clinical judgment and habit; a simple clinical method was adopted by Schamroth—in the normal individual a distinct aperture or 'window', usually diamond-shaped, is formed at the base of the nail beds; early clubbing obliterates this window.

Radiological changes occur in less than one-fifth of cases. They include phalangeal demineralization and irregular thickening of the cortical diaphysis. Ungual tufts generally show considerable variations and may be prominent in advanced stages of the disease. Atrophy may be present.

Congenital clubbed fingers may be accompanied by abnormalities and deformities such as hyperkeratosis of the palms and soles, and cortical hypertrophy of the long bones. Familial clubbing may occur in conjunction with familial, hypertrophic osteoarthropathy; some authors regard simple clubbing as a mild form of the latter. Isolated 'watch-glass' nails without their accompanying deformities are also constitutionally determined.

Very rare cases of unilateral hippocratic nails have been reported due to obstructed circulation, oedema of the soft tissues and dystrophies of the affected parts.

The pathological process which appears to be responsible for clubbing and its associated changes is hypervascularity resulting from the opening of many anastomotic shunts. In clubbed digits the nail bed may be thickened to greater than 2 mm.

Hypertrophic pulmonary osteoarthropathy

This disorder is characterized by the following five signs:

a) Clubbing of the nails.

b) Hypertrophy of the upper and lower extremities, which is similar to the deformity found in acromegaly.

c) Joint manifestations with pseudo-inflammatory, symmetrical, painful arthropathy of the large limb joints, especially those of the lower limbs. This syndrome is almost pathognomonic of malignant chest tumours, especially lung carcinoma, mesotheliomas of the pleura and less commonly bronchiectasis. Associated gynaecomastia may be found in such cases.

d) There may be bone changes due to bilateral, proliferative periostitis, with a translucent thin line between the periosteal reaction and the thickened cortex—especially over the distal ends of the long bones. Moderate, diffuse decalcification may also be present.

e) Peripheral neuro-vascular disorders such as local cyanosis and paraesthesia are not uncommon.

Hypertrophic osteoarthropathy confined to the lower extremities appears as a manifestation of arterial graft sepsis.

Pachydermoperiostosis (Figure 1.5)

Pachydermoperiostosis (idiopathic hypertrophic osteoarthropathy) is very rare. In most of the reported cases the digital changes usually begin at or about the time of puberty. The ends of the fingers and toes are bulbous and often grotesque, with hyperhidrosis of the hands and the feet. The clubbing stops abruptly at the distal interphalangeal joint. In this type the lesions of the fingertips are clinically identical to those of hypertrophic pulmonary osteoarthropathy. However, in pachydermoperiostosis there is no dividing line between the periosteal new bone and the thicken cortex, and decalcified areas do not occur. The pachydermal change of the extremities and face, with furrowing and oiliness of the skin, is the most characteristic feature of the disorder; it is described in the French literature as the Touraine, Solente and Golé syndrome.

Nevertheless, in hypertrophic pulmonary osteo-arthropathy there may be facial skin and scalp changes which are indistinguishable from those seen in pachydermoperiostosis; this could be explained by a common genetic factor. The differential diagnosis includes acromegaly, which enhances tufting of the terminal phalanges but does not cause acro-osteolysis. Thyroid acropachy is usually associated with exophthalmos, pretibial myxoedema and disturbed thyroid function.

The shell nail syndrome

This syndrome occurs in some cases of bronchiec-tasis and is similar to clubbing, but there is associated atrophy of the nail bed and the underlying bone.

The principal general causes of clubbing are shown in the box on this page, with a comprehensive list in the box on page 4.

It should be noted that only rarely will clubbing, in any of its manifestations present to a dermatologist, since in most cases it is simply one sign among many relating to the primary cause.

General causes of clubbing and pseudoclubbing	
Unilateral	Aortic/subclavian aneurysm
	Brachial plexus injury
	Trauma
Lower extremity	Arterial graft sepsis
General	
Congenital	Familial/sporadic
Pulmonary	
Cardiovascular	
Gastrointestinal	Inflammatory bowel disease
	Parasitosis
	Liver disease
	Tropical sprue
Endocrine/	Thyroid
metabolic	Malnutrition
AIDS	Secondary to pulmonary infection
Pseudo-clubbing	Yellow nail syndrome (Figure 1.6)
	Gout
	Sarcoidosis
	Osteoid osteoma
	Metastases
	Congenital abnormalities
	Chronic paronychia—severe hook nail (Figure 1.7)

Comprehensive classification of clubbing

Idiopathic forms
Hereditary and congenital forms sometimes associated with other anomalies
    Familial and genotypic pachydermoperiostosis
    Facial forms (Negroes, North Africans)
    Syndrome of pernio, periostosis and lipodystrophy

Acquired forms
Thoracic organ disorders (involved in about 80 per cent of cases of clubbing, often with the common denominator of hypoxia)
    Broncho-pulmonary diseases, especially chronic and infective bronchiectasis, abscess and cyst of the lung, pulmonary tuberculosis
    Sarcoidosis, pulmonary fibrosis, emphysema, Ayerza's syndrome, chronic pulmonary venous congestion, asthma in infancy
    Blastomycosis, pneumonia, *Pneumocystis carinii*, AIDS
Thoracic tumours (Figure 1.4)
    Primary or metastatic broncho-pulmonary cancers, pleural tumours, mediastinal tumours
    Hodgkin's disease, lymphoma, pseudo-tumour due to oesophageal dilatation
Cardio-vascular diseases
    Congenital heart disease associated with cyanosis (rarely non-cyanotic)
    Thoracic vascular malformations: stenoses and arteriovenous aneurysms
    Osler's disease (sub-acute bacterial endocarditis)
    Congestive cardiac failure
    Myxoma
    Raynaud's syndrome, erythromelalgia, Maffucci's syndrome
Disorders of the alimentary tract (5 per cent of cases)
    Oesophageal, gastric and colonic cancer
    Diseases of the small intestine
    Colonic diseases
    Amoebiasis and inflammatory states of the colon
    Ulcerative colitis
    Familial polyposis, Gardner's syndrome
    Ascariasis
    Active chronic hepatitis
    Primary or secondary cirrhoses
Endocrine origin
    Diamond's syndrome (pretibial myxoedema, exophthalmos and finger clubbing)
Haematological causes
    Primary polycythaemia or secondary polycythaemia associated with hypoxia
    Poisoning by phosphorus, arsenic, alcohol, mercury or beryllium
Hypervitaminosis A
Malnutrition, kwashiorkor
Syringomyelia
Lupus erythematosus
Unilateral or limited to a few digits
    Subluxation of the shoulder (with paralysis of the brachial plexus), median nerve neuritis
    Pancoast–Tobias' syndrome
    Aneurysm of the aorta or the subclavian artery
    Sarcoidosis
    Tophaceous gout
Lower extremities
    Arterial graft sepsis
Isolated forms
    Local injury, whitlow, lymphangitis
    Subungual epidermoid inclusions
Transitory form
    Physiological in the newborn child (due to reversal of the circulation at birth)
Occupational acro-osteolysis (exposure to vinyl chloride)

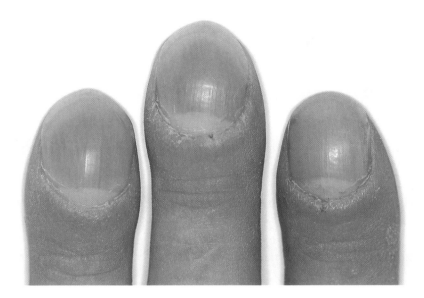

Figure 1.1 Clubbing of fingers.

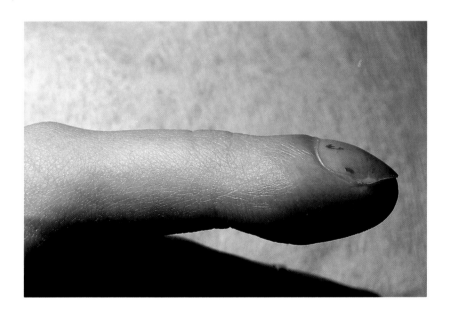

Figure 1.2 Clubbing of fingers—lateral view showing fusiform swelling.

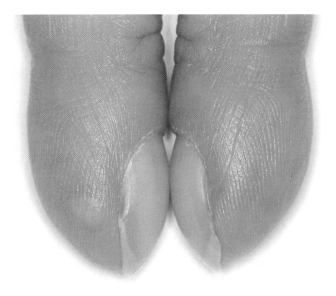

Figure 1.3   Clubbing of fingers—demonstrating typical nail curvature.

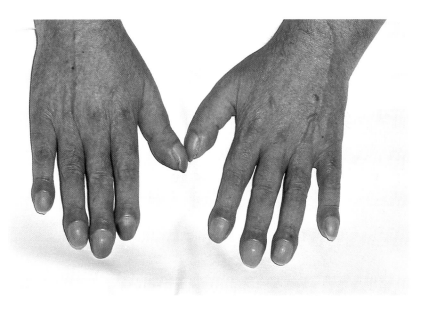

Figure 1.4   Hands showing uniform clubbing of all digits due to carcinoma of the lung.

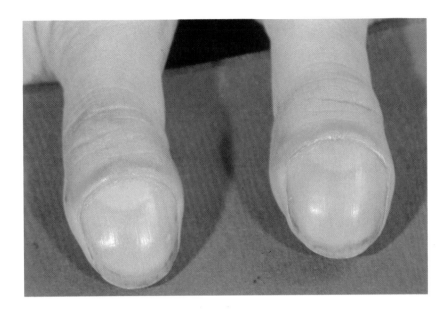

Figure 1.5 'Clubbing' of pachydermoperiostitis.

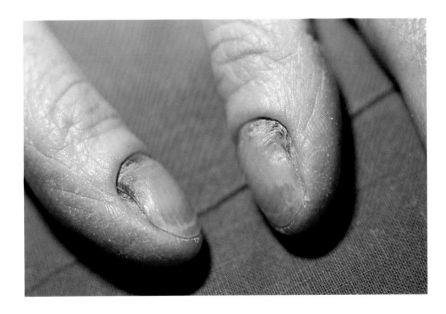

Figure 1.6 Pseudoclubbing of fingers in yellow nail syndrome; the nail itself is curved but the digit is otherwise normal.

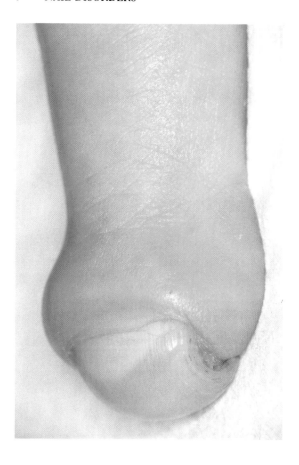

Figure 1.7 Pseudoclubbing related to hook nail deformity.

Koilonychia (Spoon-shaped nails) (Figures 1.8–1.13)

This sign is the opposite of clubbing which is an exaggeration of the normal curvature of the nail, the latter reflecting the shape of the terminal phalanx. (The nail is firmly attached to bone by vertical dermal connective tissue bundles in the subungual area which bond directly to the bony periosteum.)

In the early stages of koilonychia there is flattening of the nail plate. Later, the edges become everted upwards and the nail appears concave—thus the descriptive term 'spoon nail'. In mild cases the water test may enable a drop of water to be retained on the nail plate. The subungual tissues may be normal, or affected by hyperkeratosis at the lateral and/or the distal margin.

The main types of koilonychia are:

● In neonates and in infancy koilonychia it is a temporary physiological condition (Figure 1.10). There is proven correlation between koilonychia and iron deficiency (with normal haemoglobin values) in infants.

● Koilonychia is a common manifestation of the rare Plummer–Vinson syndrome in association with anaemia, dysphagia and glossitis.

When subungual keratosis accompanies koilonychia, psoriasis should be considered, as should occupational causes such as in cement workers, constant oil immersion in car mechanics, and so on.

● Thin nails of any cause (old age, peripheral arterial disease and so on) (Figure 1.11).

● Soft nails of any cause (mainly occupational) (Figure 1.12).

● Hereditary and congenital forms associated with other nail anomalies such as leukonychia.

Commonest causes of koilonychia	
Physiological	Early childhood (Figure 1.10)
Idiopathic	
Congenital	LEOPARD syndrome
	Ectodermal dysplasias
	Trichothiodystrophy
	Nail–patella syndrome
Acquired	
Metabolic/endocrine	Iron deficiency (Figures 1.8 and 1.9)
	Haemochromatosis
	Porphyria
	Renal dialysis/transplant
	Thyroid disease
	Acromegaly
Dermatoses	Psoriasis
	Lichen planus (Figure 1.13)
	Alopecia areata
	Darier's disease
	Raynaud's syndrome
Occupational	Contact with oils, eg engineering industry (Figure 1.12)
Infections	Onychomycosis
	Syphilis
Traumatic	Toes of rickshaw boys
Carpal tunnel syndrome	

The commonest presentations of koilonychia are probably occupational softening (Figure 1.12) and iron deficiency (Figures 1.8–1.9). The box lists most of the well-known causes.

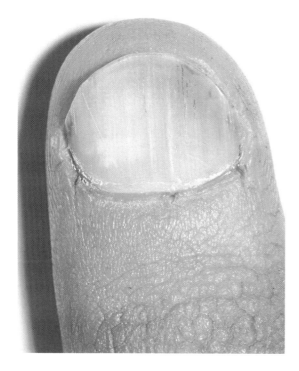

Figure 1.8 Koilonychia.

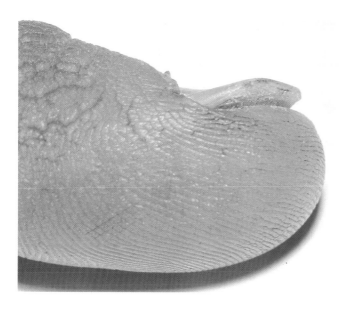

Figure 1.9 Koilonychia—lateral view showing inverse curvature of the nail.

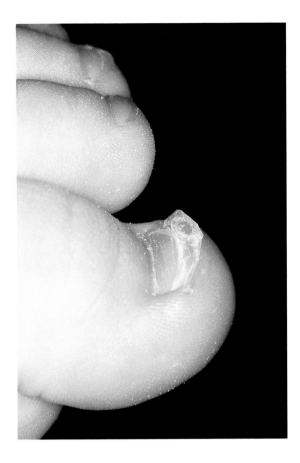

Figure 1.10 Physiological koilonychia in early childhood; this reverts to 'normal' curvature as the nail thickens.

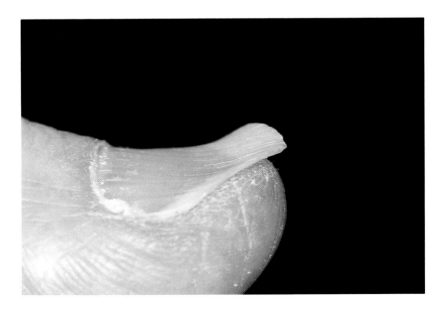

Figure 1.11 Koilonychia—thin nail type; any cause of thin nail plate may cause this.

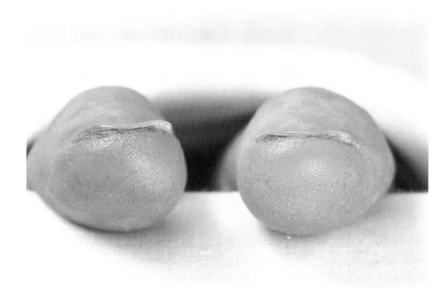

Figure 1.12 Distal view of koilonychia due to occupational contact with motor oils.

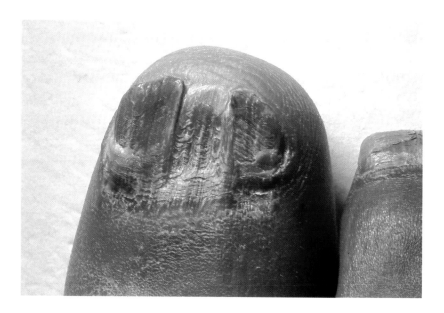

Figure 1.13 Lichen planus dystrophy showing koilonychia of residual nail plate.

Transverse overcurvature (Figures 1.14–1.20)

There are three main types of this condition: the arched, pincer and trumpet nail; the tile-shaped nail; and a third less common variety, the 'plicatured' nail (Diagram 1.1).

Pincer nail

Pincer nail is a dystrophy characterized by transverse overcurvature that increases along the longitudinal axis of the nail and reaches its greatest proportion at the distal part (Figure 1.14). At this point, the lateral borders tighten around the soft tissues which are pinched without necessarily breaking through the epidermis. After a while, the soft tissue may actually disappear and this may be accompanied by resorption of the underlying bone. A subungual exostosis may present in this way: the dorsal extension of bone produces a pincer nail—the exostosis must be excised. The lateral borders of the nail exert a constant pressure, permanently constricting the deformed nail plate. In extreme cases, they may joint together, forming a tunnel; or they may roll about themselves, taking the form of a cone. In certain varieties, the nails are shaped like claws, sometimes resembling pachyonychia congenita.

This morphological abnormality would be no more than a curiosity if the constriction were not occasionally accompanied by pain which is sometimes provoked by the lightest of touch, such as the weight of a bedsheet. The origin of this dystrophy probably resides in a developmental anomaly and may be inherited. Some cases have been attributed to wearing ill-fitting shoes. Underlying pathology, such as subungual exostosis in the toes and inflammatory osteoarthritis, should always be looked for, especially if the fingers are involved.

Tile-shaped nail

The tile-shaped nail presents with an increase in the transverse curvature; the lateral edges of the nail remain parallel (Figure 1.15).

Plicatured nail

In the plicatured variety the surface of the nail plate is almost flat, while one or both lateral margins are sharply angled, forming vertical sides which are parallel (Figure 1.16).

Although these deformities may be associated with ingrowing nails, inflammatory oedema due to the constriction of the soft tissues is unusual.

Transverse overcurvature	
Congenital	Hidrotic ectodermal dysplasia (Figure 1.18)
	Hypohidrotic ectodermal dysplasia (Figure 1.19)
	Congenital onychodysplasia of index fingernails
	Yellow nail syndrome
Developmental	Pincer nails (Figures 1.14 and 1.19)
Acquired	Osteoarthritis (Figure 1.17)
	Neglect, eg toe nails in old age (Figure 1.17)

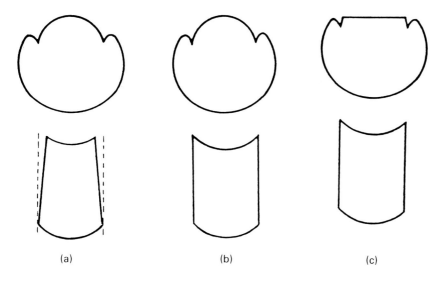

(a)   (b)   (c)

Diagram 1.1   Transverse overcurvature showing the three sub-types: (a) pincer or trumpet nail, (b) tile-shaped nail and (c) plicatured nail with sharply angled lateral margins.

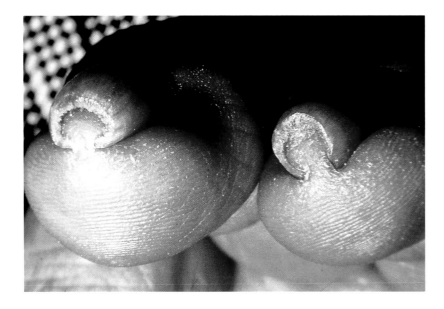

Figure 1.14   Finger pincer nail deformity.

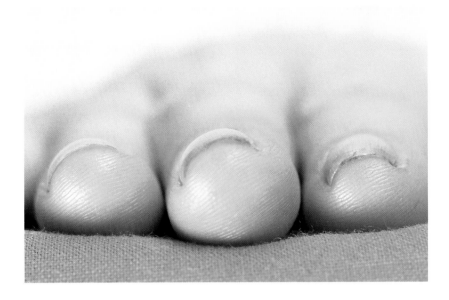

Figure 1.15 Tile-shaped overcurvature—here due to early yellow nail syndrome.

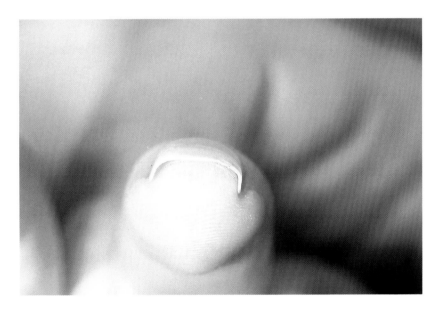

Figure 1.16 Bilateral plicatured overcurvature: may cause finger nail 'ingrowing'.

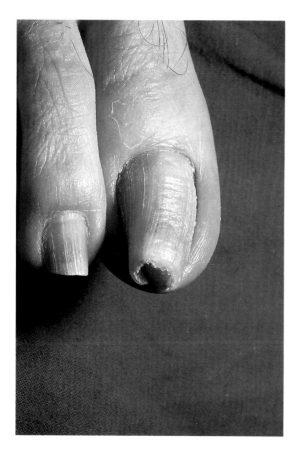

Figure 1.17 'Trumpet nail' deformity—here related to old age, neglect and osteoarthritis.

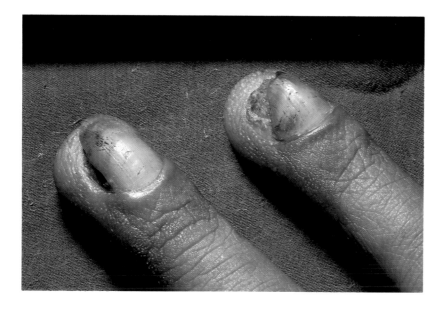

Figure 1.18 Transverse overcurvature in hidrotic ectodermal dysplasia.

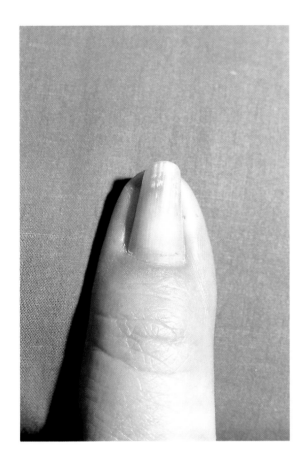

Figure 1.19 Increased transverse overcurvature (almost pincer nail) in hypohidrotic ectodermal dysplasia.

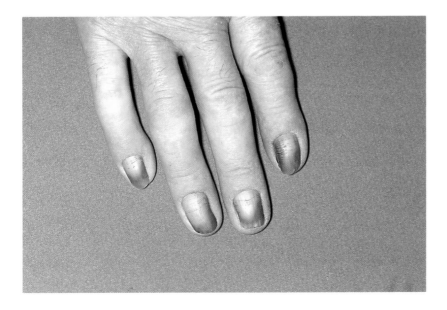

Figure 1.20 Overcurvature (and thickening of nails) in yellow nail syndrome.

Dolichonychia (Long nails) (Figures 1.21–1.22)

In this condition the length of the nail is much greater than the width. It has been described in:

- Ehlers–Danlos syndrome

- Marfan's syndrome

- Eunuchoidism

- Hypopituitarism

- Hypohidrotic ectodermal dysplasia (Figure 1.22)

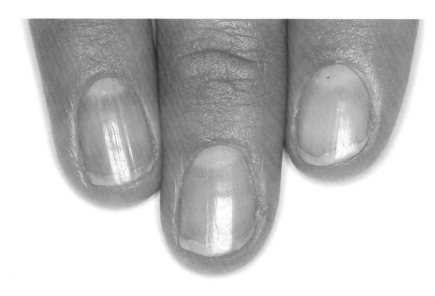

Figure 1.21   Dolichonychia.

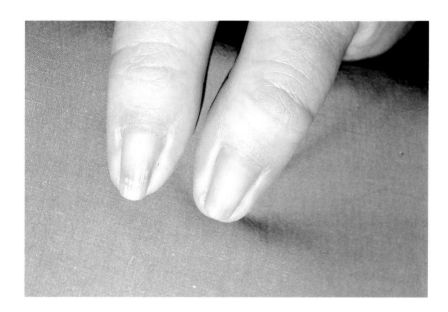

Figure 1.22   Hypohidrotic ectodermal dysplasia with long narrow nails (overcurving).

Brachyonychia (Short nails) (Figures 1.23–1.30)

In this condition, the width of the nail plate (and the nail bed) is greater than the length. It may occur in isolation or associated with a shortening of the terminal phalanx. The 'racquet thumb' is usually inherited as an autosomal dominant trait (Figure 1.24). All the fingers may be involved. The epiphyses of the terminal phalanx of the thumb are normally closing at the age of 13–14 in girls and slightly later in boys. In individuals with this hereditary defect the epiphyseal line is obliterated on the affected side at the age of 7–10 years, while it is still present according to age in the normal thumb. Since the periosteal growth continues the result will be the deformed racquet-like thumb. Racquet nails have been reported in association with brachydactylia and multiple malignant Spiegler tumours. A syndrome of broad thumbs, broad great toes, facial abnormalities and mental retardation has been described.

The box on this page lists many well-recognized causes of short nails whilst the box on page 21 gives details of the rarer hereditary and congenital conditions in which it occurs.

Brachyonychia		
Congenital	Isolated defect: racquet thumb (Figures 1.23, 1.24)	
	Rubenstein–Taybi: 'broad thumbs' syndrome (Figure 1.25)	
	Micronychia with trisomy 21	
	Congenital malalignment—great toe nails (Figure 1.26)	
Acquired	Nail biters (Figure 1.27)	
	Associated with bone resorption in hyperparathyroidism (Figures 1.28, 1.29)	
	Psoriatic arthropathy (Figure 1.30)	

Hereditary forms of broad nails (some also with pseudoclubbing)

Inheritances are indicated as follows:

AD autosomal dominant   AR autosomal recessive   XD sex-linked dominant   XR sex-linked recessive

Diseases	Inheritance	Clinical features
Acrocephalosyndactyly	AD	Craniosynostosis. Syndactyly. Ankylosis and other skeletal deformities
Acrodysostosis	AD	Fingernails short, broad and oval in shape. Short fingers. Nasal and midface hypoplasia. Mental retardation. Growth failure. Pigmented naevi
Berk–Tabatznik syndrome	?	Stub thumb, short terminal phalanges of all fingers except dig V. Bilateral optic atrophy, cervical kyphosis
Familial mandibuloacral dysplasia	AR	Club-shaped terminal phalanges. Mandibular hypoplasia, delayed cranial closure. Dysplastic clavicles. Atrophy of skin over hands and feet. Alopecia
Keipert syndrome	AR or XR	Unusual facies with large nose. Protruded upper lip. Short and broad distal phalanges of halluces and fingers, except dig V
Larsen's syndrome	AR or AD	Stub thumbs, cylindrical fingers, flattened peculiar facies, widespread eyes. Multiple dislocations, short metacarpals
Nanocephalic dwarfism	AR	Low birth weight with adult head circumference. Mental retardation. Beak-like protrusion of nose. Multiple osseous anomalies. Clubbing of fingers
Otopalatodigital syndrome	XR or AR	Broad, short nails especially of thumbs and big toes. Mental retardation. Prominent occiput. Hypoplasia of facial bones. Cloven palate. Conductive deafness
Pleonosteosis	?	Short stature. Spade-like hands with thick palmar pads. Massive knobby thumbs. Short flexed fingers. Limited joint motion with contractures
Pseudohypoparathyroidism, hereditary osteodystrophy	XD or AR	Short stature. Round face. Depressed nasal bridge. Short metacarpals. Mental retardation. Cataracts in 25 per cent. Enamel hypoplasia. Calcifications in skin
Puretic syndrome		Osteolysis of peripheral phalanges. Stunted growth. Contracture of joints. Multiple subcutaneous nodes, atrophic sclerodermic skin
Rubinstein–Taybi syndrome (Figure 1.25)	AD	Broad thumb with radial angulation and great toes. High palate, short stature, mental retardation, peculiar facies
Spiegler tumours and racquet nails	?	Brachydactyly. Turban tumours
Stub thumb with racquet nail (Figure 1.24)	AD	No other defects. Appears at the age of 7–10 by early obliteration of the epiphyseal line

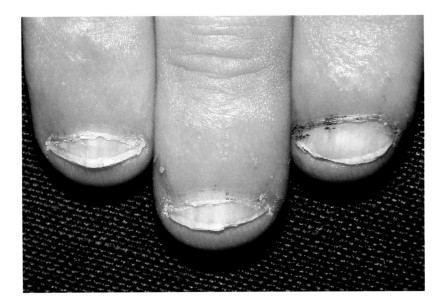

Figure 1.23   Brachyonychia.

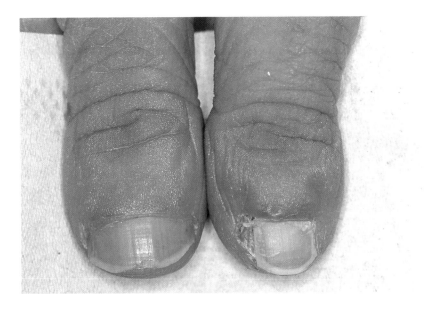

Figure 1.24   Racquet nail deformity of thumbs (the nail on the right shows surgical narrowing).

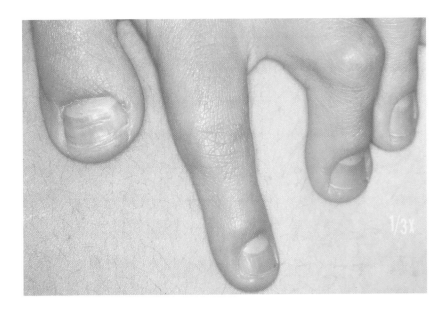

Figure 1.25 Brachyonychia in Rubinstein–Taybi syndrome (courtesy of Dr Roger and Prof Souteyrand, Clermont-Ferrand.)

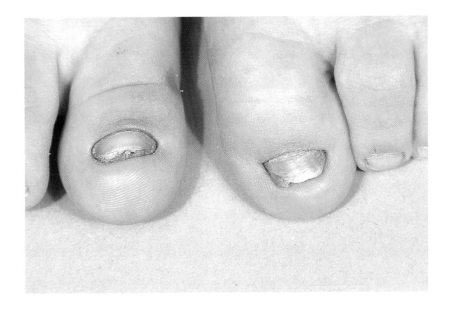

Figure 1.26 Short nails in congenital malalignment of great toe nails (Baran syndrome). (See also Figure 7.2.)

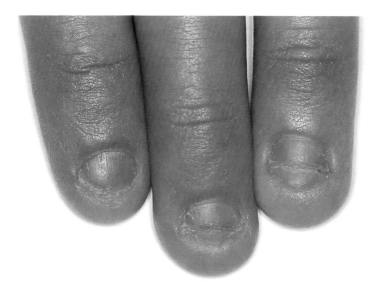

Figure 1.27 Persistent short nails due to nail biting.

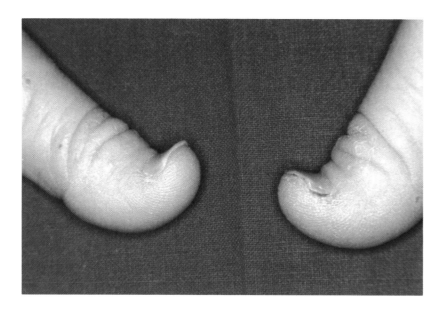

Figure 1.28 Short nails due to hyperparathyroidism (haemodialysis patient). (Courtesy of Dr Schubert, Mulhouse.)

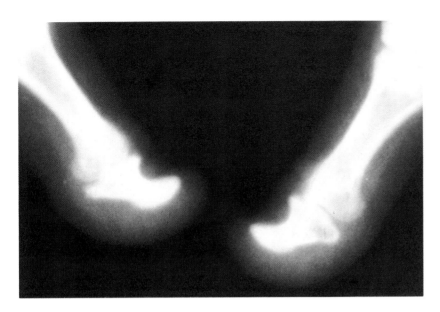

Figure 1.29   X-ray of digits seen in Figure 1.28.

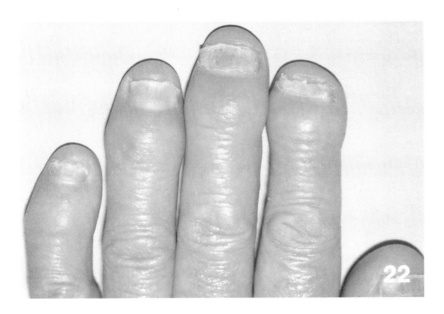

Figure 1.30   Short nails associated with psoriatic arthropathy.

Parrot beak nails (Figures 1.31–1.32)

In this symmetrical overcurvature of the free edge, some finger nails mimic the beak of a parrot; this shape disappears temporarily in soaking the nails in lukewarm water for about half an hour. No abnormality may be noted clinically as such patients usually trim their nails close to the line of separation from the nail bed.

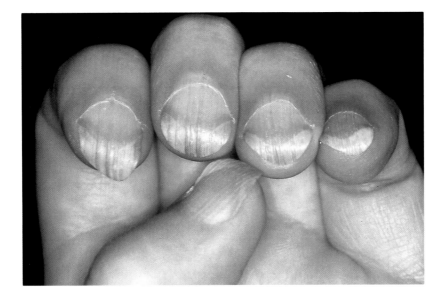

Figure 1.31 Parrot beak deformity—usually cut short and not visible.

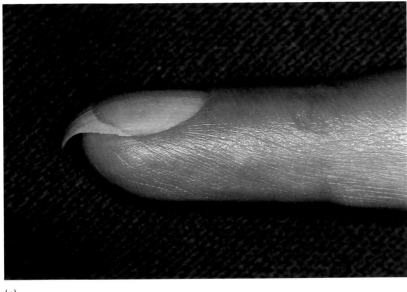

(a)

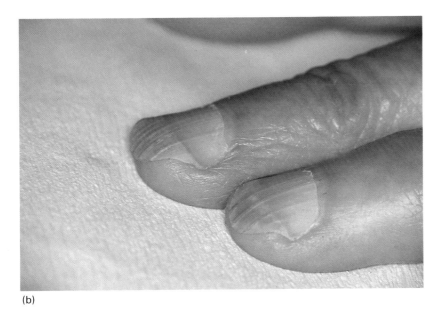

(b)

Figure 1.32 Lateral view of parrot beak deformity.

Hook and claw-like nails (Figures 1.33–1.36)

One or both little toe nails are often rounded like a claw. This condition predominates in women wearing high heels and narrow shoes and is often associated with the development of hyperkeratosis such as calluses on the feet. Congenital claw-like fingers and toe nails have been reported. Claw nails may be curved dorsally showing a concave upper surface, resembling onychogryphosis or post-traumatic hook nail (Figures 1.33, 1.34). In the nail-patella syndrome when the pointed lunula sign occurs, if the nail is not manicured it will tend to grow with a pointed tip and may resemble a claw (Figure 1.36).

Hook-shaped nails may be an isolated defect—congenital or acquired (eg traumatic) (Figures 1.33, 1.34).

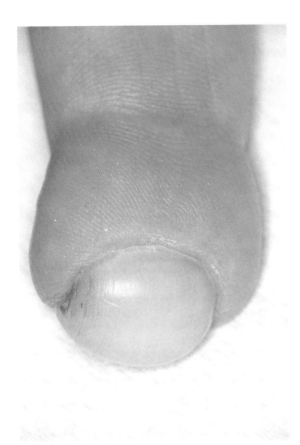

Figure 1.33 Hook-shaped deformity.

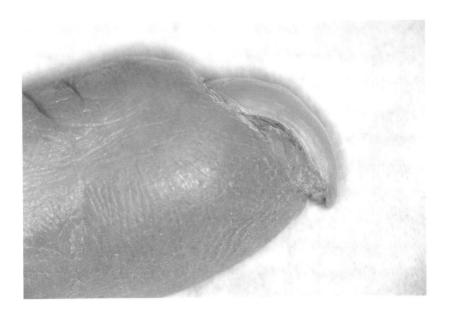

Figure 1.34 Lateral view of digit seen in Figure 1.33.

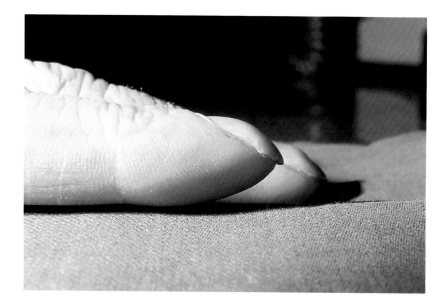

Figure 1.35   Normal nail—beak/early hook deformity (normally cut shorter).

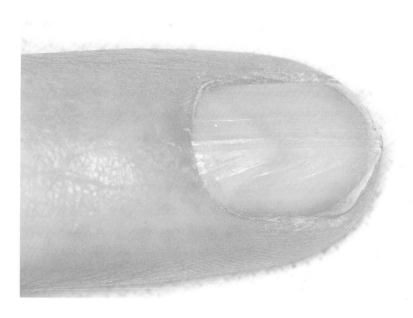

Figure 1.36   Nail–patella syndrome—pointed lunula, gives pointed (almost claw-like) nail if not cut short as shown here.

Micro- and macronychia (Figures 1.37–1.42)

In macronychia the nails involving one or more digits are wider than normal, with nail bed and matrix being similarly affected. They may occur as an isolated defect or in association with megadactyly as in von Recklinghausen's disease and epiloia (Figure 1.38).

In Iso–Kikuchi (COIF) syndrome there are two types of micronychia. The most frequent is medially sited. In 'rolled' micronychia the nail is centrally located (Figures 1.39, 1.40).

Overlapping of the nail surface by enlarged lateral nail fold may result in apparent micronychia.

The box below lists the known associations.

Micro and macronychia

Congenital	Ectodermal dysplasias (Figure 1.42) Congenital onchodysplasia of index finger nails (Figures 1.39, 1.40) Dyskeratosis congenita Chromosomal abnormalities Nail–patella syndrome

Acquired	Fetal teratogens
	  Hydantoins
	  Alcohol
	  Warfarin
	Amniotic bands

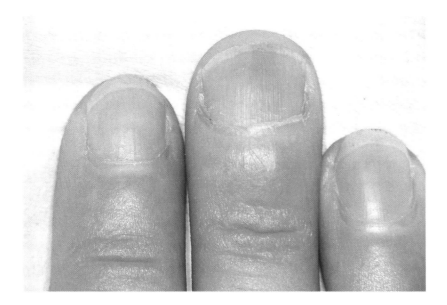

Figure 1.37   Macronychia of middle finger.

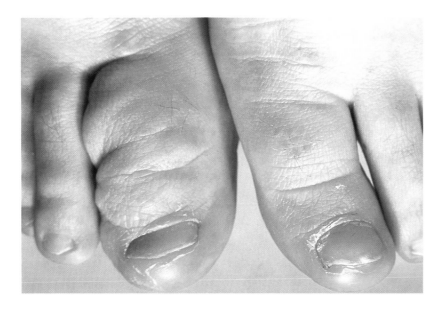

Figure 1.38   Megadactyly and macronychia associated with von Recklinghausen's multiple neurofibromatosis.

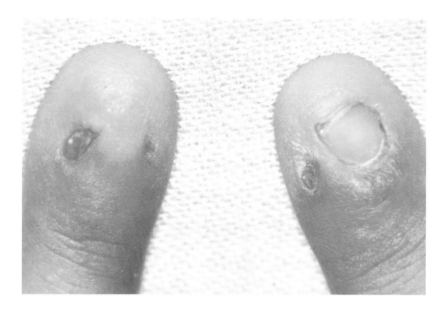

Figure 1.39 Micronychia in congenital onychodysplasia of index finger nails (courtesy of Prof A Claudy, Saint-Etienne).

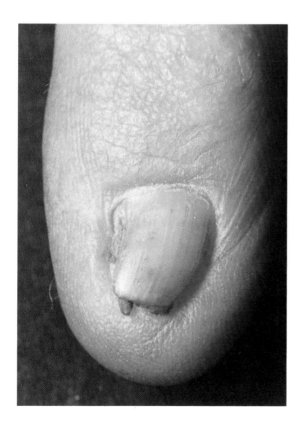

Figure 1.40 'Rolled' micronychia in congenital onychodysplasia of index finger nails.

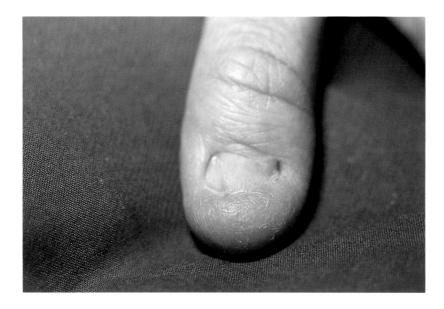

Figure 1.41 Micronychia in nail–patella syndrome.

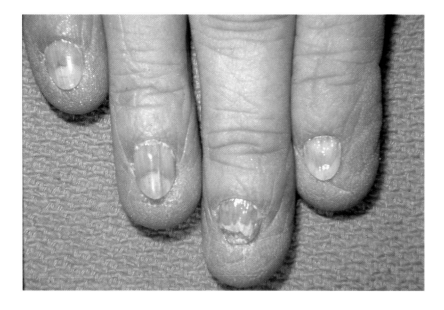

Figure 1.42 Hidrotic ectodermal dysplasis—micronychia with onycholysis (courtesy of Prof L Norton, Boston).

Worn down and shiny nails (Figures 1.43–1.44)

Patients with atopic dermatitis or chronic erythroderma may be 'chronic scratchers and rubbers'. The surface of the nail plate becomes glossy and shiny and the free edge is worn away. *Usure des ongles* may also occur in many different manual occupations. This condition has recently been described as a particular occupational hazard of individuals handling heavy, plastic bags.

Worn down nails

Occupational causes

| Smooth shiny nails | Atopic eczema Pruritic lymphoma Chronic pruritis | (Figure 1.43) |

| Distal fraying | Trauma Darier's disease (Figure 1.44) Old age Nail scratchers |

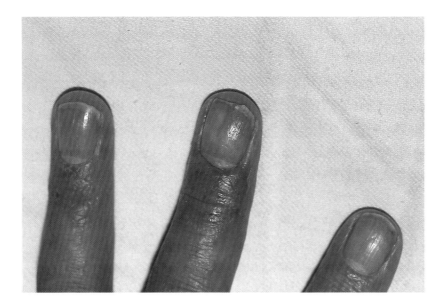

Figure 1.43 Shiny nails due to 'rubbing'—associated pruritic eruptions.

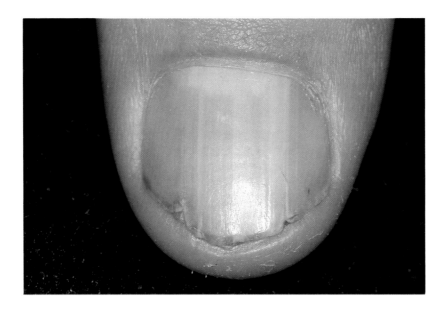

Figure 1.44 Darier's disease—worn down tips due to intrinsic keratinization defect; note associated white lines.

Anonychia and onychatrophy (Figures 1.45–1.55)

It is quite impossible to differentiate completely these two signs in the light of current knowledge. In principle the term 'anonychia' (total or partial) is probably best reserved for conditions in which the nail has failed to develop; 'onychatrophy' should be used to describe processes in which the nail has initially formed satisfactorily and then shown total or partial regression.

In aplastic anonychia, a rare congenital disorder occasionally associated with other defects such as ectrodactyly, the nail never forms. Loose horny masses are produced by the metaplastic, squamous epithelium of the matrix and the nail bed in anonychia keratodes. Hypoplasia of the nail plates is a hallmark of the nail–patella syndrome; in the least-affected cases only the ulnar half of each thumb nail is missing.

Onychatrophy presents as a reduction in size and thickness of the nail plate, often accompanied by fragmentation and splitting, for example in lichen planus (Figures 1.48–1.50). This condition may progressively worsen, scar tissue eventually replacing the atrophic nail plate. The box below shows the commoner known causes of anonychia and onychatrophy.

Anonychia (Figures 1.45–1.47)

Permanent hypo- or anonychia
  +/− ectrodactyly
  +/− dental malformations
  Nail–patella syndrome
  Congenital onychodysplasia of index fingernails
  Coffin–Siris syndrome with many congenital defects, eg DOOR syndrome (deafness, onycho-osteodystrophy, mental retardation)

Onychatrophy (Figures 1.48–1.55)

With pterygium (Figure 1.48)
  Lichen planus (Figures 1.48–1.50)
  Acrosclerosis (Figure 1.51)
  Onychotillomania (Figure 1.52)
  Lesch–Nyhan
  Chronic graft versus host disease
  Stevens–Johnson or Lyell syndrome
  Cicatricial pemphigoid (Figure 1.53)

Without pterygium
  Severe paronychia with nail dystrophy
  Stevens–Johnson or Lyell syndrome
  Epidermolysis bullosa (Figure 1.54)
  Amyloid
  Etretinate nail dystrophy (Figure 1.55)
  Idiopathic atrophy of childhood
  Severe psoriatic nail dystrophy

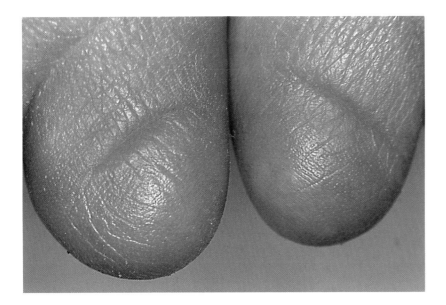

Figure 1.45   Congenital absence of nails.

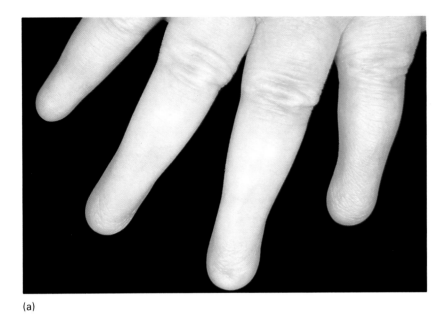

(a)

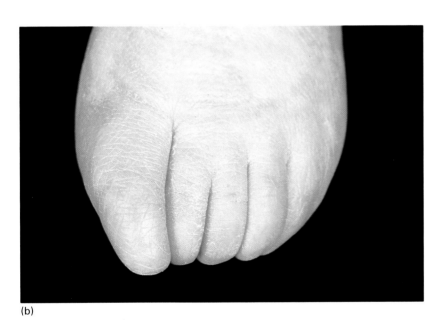

(b)

Figure 1.46   Absence of nails in DOOR syndrome (courtesy of Prof Nevin, Royal Victoria Hospital, Belfast).

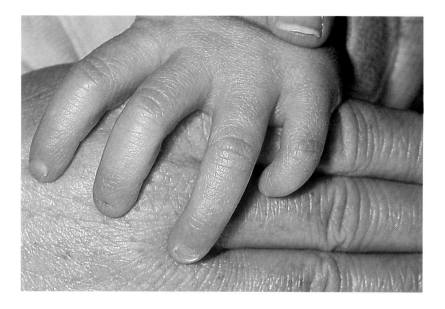

Figure 1.47   Congenital absence of nail—isolated defect.

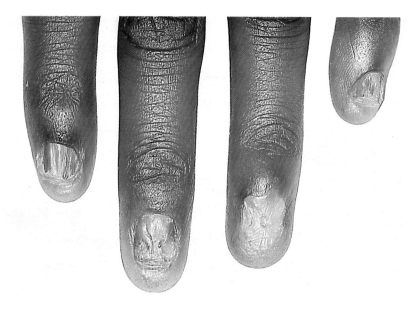

Figure 1.48   Nail atrophy in childhood, nail lichen planus; pterygium-type scarring is present.

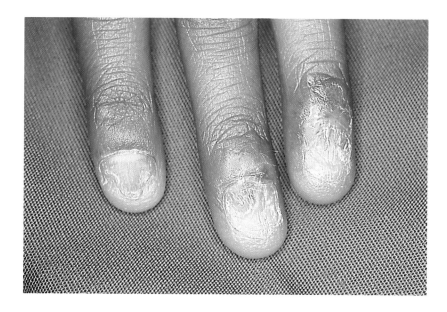

Figure 1.49 Lichen planus atrophic—more severe than in Figure 1.48, with proximal nail fold lichen planus visible.

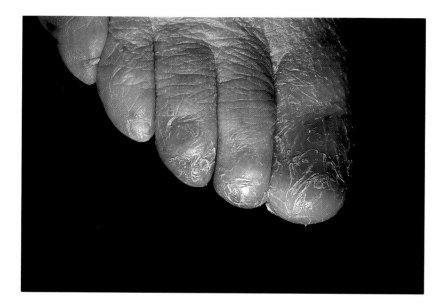

Figure 1.50 Total nail atrophy in lichen planus (erosive type).

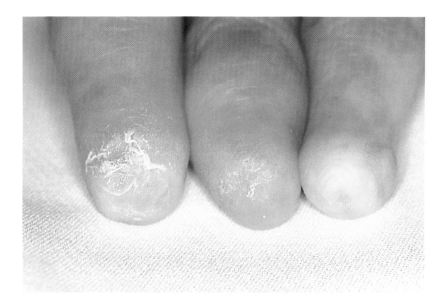

Figure 1.51 Anonychia in severe acrosclerosis (scleroderma).

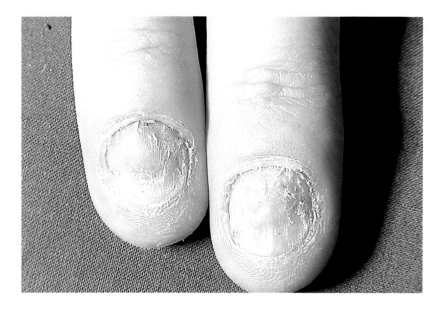

Figure 1.52 Nail atrophy in onychotillomania.

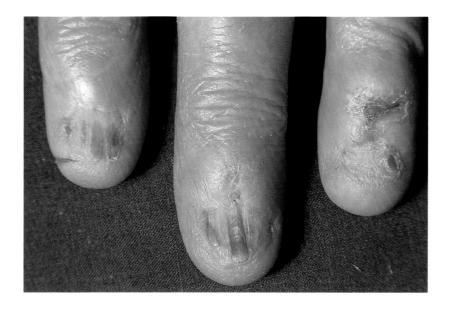

Figure 1.53   Nail atrophy in cicatricial pemphigoid.

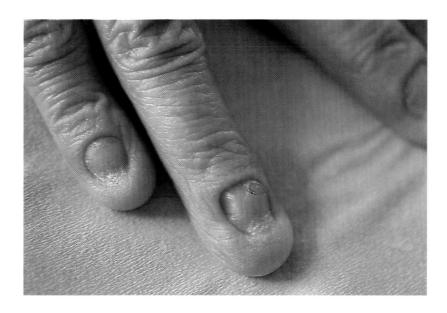

Figure 1.54   Nail atrophy in epidermolysis bullosa.

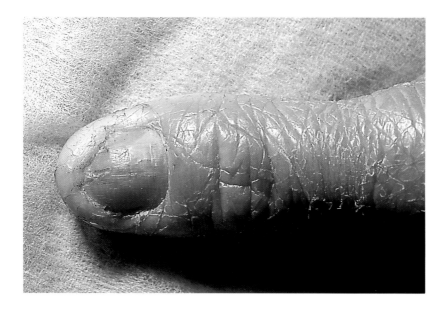

Figure 1.55   Atrophic nails due to the retinoid etretinate.

Further reading

Clubbing

Dickinson CJ and **Martin JF,** Megakaryocytes and platelet clumps as the cause of finger clubbing. *Lancet* (1987) **ii**:1434–5.

Fischer DS, Singer DH and **Feldman SM,** Clubbing, a review, with emphasis on hereditary acropachy. *Medicine* (1964) **43**:459–79.

Koilonychia

Stone OJ, Clubbing and koilonychia. *Dermatol Clin* (1985) **3**:485–90.

Hogan GR and **Jones B,** The relationship between koilonychia and iron deficiency in infants. *J Pediatr* (1970) **77**:1054–7.

Transverse overcurvature

Cornelius CE and **Shelley WB,** Pincer nail syndrome. *Arch Surg* (1968) **96**:321–2.

Brachyonychia

Rubinstein JH, The broad thumbs syndrome—progress report 1968. *Birth Defects: Original Article Series* (1969) **V**(2):25–41.

Micro- and macronychia

Kikuchi I, Congenital polyonychias: reduction versus duplication digit malformations. *Int J Dermatol* (1985) **24**:211–15.

Telfer NR, Barth JH and **Dawber RPR,** Congenital and hereditary nail dystrophies—an embryological approach to classification. *Clin Exp Dermatol* (1988) **13**:160–3.

Anonychia and nail atrophy

Zaias N, The nail in lichen planus. *Arch Dermatol* (1970) **101**:264–71.

2

Modifications of nail surface

Longitudinal lines (Figures 2.1–2.10)

Longitudinal lines, or striations, may appear as indented grooves or projecting ridges.

Longitudinal grooves

Longitudinal grooves represent long-lasting abnormalities and can occur under the following conditions:

a) Physiological, as shallow and delicate furrows, usually parallel, and separated by low, projecting ridges. They become more prominent with age and in certain pathological states, such as lichen planus, rheumatoid arthritis, peripheral circulatory disorders, Darier's disease and other genetic abnormalities (Figures 2.1–2.4, 2.8, 2.9).

b) Onychorrhexis is a series of narrow, longitudinal, parallel superficial furrows which have the appearance of having been scratched by an awl. Sometimes dust becomes ingrained on the nail surface. Splitting of the free edge is common.

c) Tumours, such as myxoid cysts and warts, located in the proximal nail fold area, may exert pressure on the nail matrix and produce a wide, deep, longitudinal groove or canal, which will disappear if the cause is removed.

d) Median nail dystrophy (Figures 2.6–2.7). This uncommon condition consists of a longitudinal defect of the thumb nails in the mid-line or just off centre, starting at the cuticle and growing out of the free edge. It may be associated with an enlarged lunula. In early descriptions, the base of the 2 to 5 mm wide groove with steep edges showed numerous transverse defects. More recent reports have shown longitudinal fissures as 'dystrophia longitudinalis fissuriformis'. In some cases median longitudinal ridges have been observed, occasionally combined with fissures and/or a groove, developed from the distal edge of the nail plate to the matrix. Often a few short feathery cracks, chevron-shaped, extend laterally from the split. The so-called 'naevus striatus symmetricus of the thumbs' corresponds to this form. Median nail dystrophy is usually symmetrical and most often affects both thumbs. Sometimes other fingers are involved, seldom the toes (usually the big toe). After several months or years, the nail returns to normal but recurrences are not exceptional. Familial cases have been recorded. In all cases the aetiology is unknown but it has been suggested that the deformity is usually due to self-inflicted trauma resulting from a tic or habit.

Treatment of recalcitrant cases may be identical to the tic of pushing back the cuticle.

e) A central longitudinal depression is found in

'washboard nail plates' caused by chronic, mechanical injury. Unlike median nail dystrophy (Heller's dystrophy), the cuticle is pushed back and there is accompanying inflammation of the proximal nail fold. Splits due to trauma, or those occurring in the nail–patella syndrome and in pterygium, are generally obvious. Longitudinal splits may also result from Raynaud's disease, lichen striatus and trachyonychia.

Nail wrapping (Chapter 9) may reduce the disability produced by the fissure. The proximal nail fold must be protected from repeated minor trauma.

Longitudinal ridges

Small rectilinear projections extend from the proximal nail fold as far as the free edge of the nail; or they may stop short. They may be interrupted at regular intervals, giving rise to a beaded appearance. Sometimes a wide, longitudinal median ridge has the appearance, in cross-section, of a circumflex accent. This condition is inherited and affects mainly the thumb and index fingers of both hands.

The following box shows the principal causes of longitudinal lines and grooves.

Causes of longitudinal lines

Coloured lines

White	See leukonychia (pages 146–54)
Black	See melanonychia (pages 155–60)
Red	Darier's disease (Figure 2.4)
	Vascular tumours
	Glomus (Figure 2.10)
	Cirsoid

Linear ridges

Single	Familial
	Median canaliform dystrophy (Figures 2.6, 2.7)
	Trauma (isolated or repeated)
	Tumours
Multiple	Normal—increase with age after early adulthood (Figures 2.1–2.3)
	With all causes of thin nail plates
	Lichen planus (Figure 2.9)
	Rheumatoid arthritis
	Graft versus host disease
	Psoriasis
	Darier's disease
	Poor circulation
	Collagen vascular disorders
	Radiation
	Frostbite
	Alopecia areata
	Nail–patella syndrome

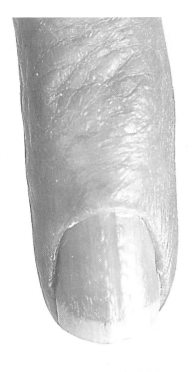

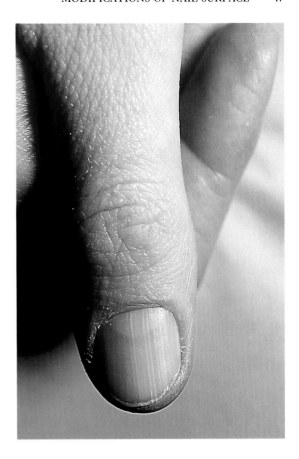

Figure 2.1 Age-related longitudinal lines—normal subject aged 65 years.

Figure 2.2 Normal longitudinal lines—subject aged 56 years.

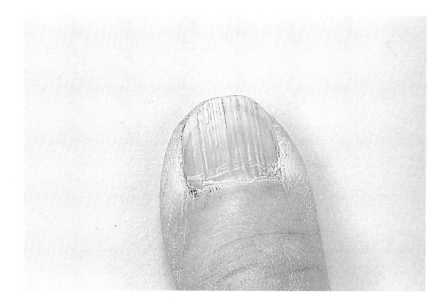

Figure 2.3   Old-age longitudinal lines—associated with ragged cuticle.

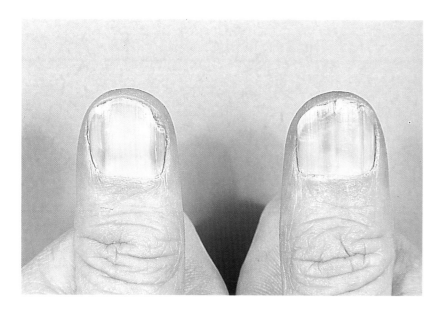

Figure 2.4   Red lines in Darier's disease.

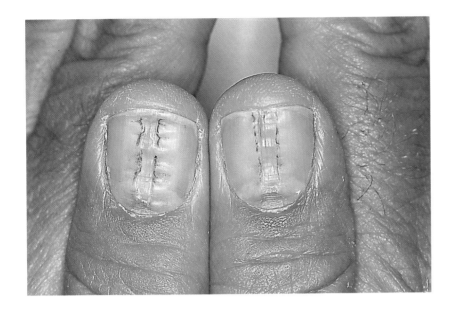

Figure 2.5 Self-induced longitudinal grooves/lines of thumb nails.

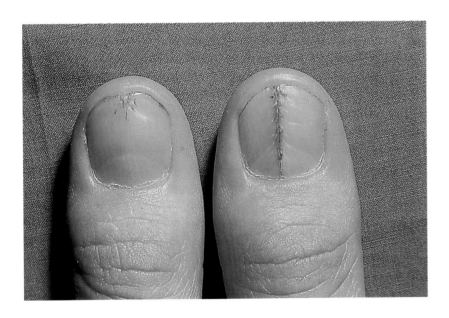

Figure 2.6 Median canaliform dystrophy (Heller's dystrophy).

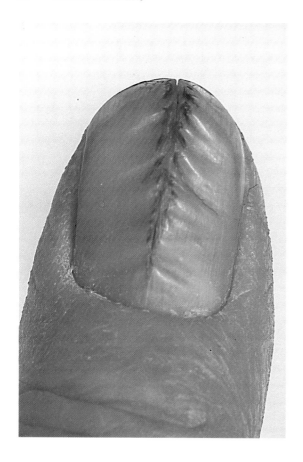

Figure 2.7   Median canaliform dystrophy—'fir-tree' deformation.

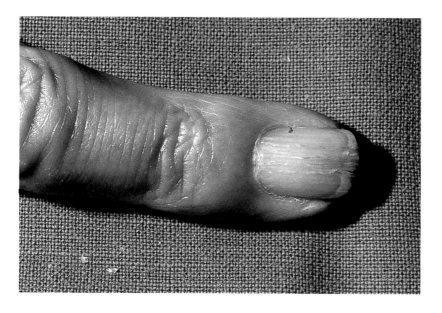

Figure 2.8   Longitudinal lines in lichen planus.

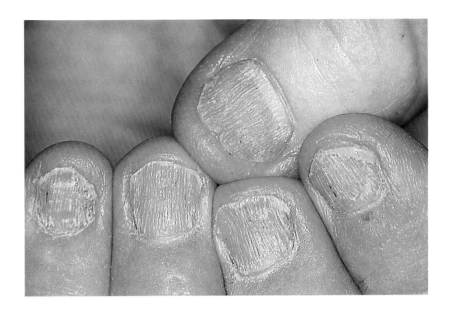

Figure 2.9 Lichen planus—longitudinal lines, nail thinning and trachyonychia ('sand-papered nails'; see pages 61–3).

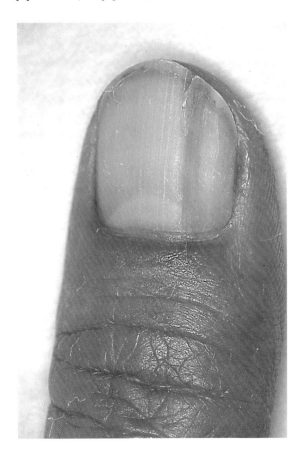

Figure 2.10 Longitudinal red line—single one due to glomus tumour.

Transverse lines (Figures 2.11–2.15)

Transverse band-like depressions extending from one lateral edge of the nail to the other and affecting all nails at corresponding levels, are called Beau's lines (Figure 2.11). They may be noted after any severe, sudden febrile attack. In milder cases the nails of the thumb and the big toe are the most reliable markers, as the former would supply information for the previous 6 months and the latter would show evidence of disease for 18 months (relating to the different rates of linear nail growth).

The width of the transverse groove represents the exact duration of the disease which has affected the matrix. The distal limit of the furrow, if abrupt, would indicate a sudden attack of disease; if sloping a more protracted onset. In fact the proximal limit of the depression may be abrupt and both limits may well be sloped.

If the duration of the disease can inhibit the activity of the matrix for 1–2 weeks for example, the transverse depression will result in a total division of the nail plate, a defect known as 'onychomadesis'. As the nail adheres firmly to the nail bed the onychomadesis remains latent for several weeks before leading to temporary shedding.

Transverse furrows may be due to measles in childhood, zinc deficiency (often multiple), Stevens–Johnson and Lyell's syndromes, cytotoxic drugs and many other non-specific events.

Beau's lines may also be physiological marks appearing with each menstrual cycle. They are also present in 92 per cent of 8- to 9-week-old normal babies.

When only few digits are involved this may indicate trauma, carpal tunnel syndrome, chronic paronychia or chronic eczema. As a consequence of a chronic condition, the lines are often numerous and curvilinear. When a series of transverse grooves parallels the proximal nail fold the cause is likely to be repeated trauma from over-zealous manicuring. Rhythmic parallel transverse grooves may be an isolated sign of psoriasis, equivalent of patterned pitting.

A nervous habit of pushing back the cuticle usually affects the thumbs which are damaged by the index finger nail of the corresponding hand: symmetrical involvement of the thumbs is the rule (Figures 2.13, 2.14) but ocasionally only one thumb is affected; or rarely, other digits may be involved, the thumb reversing roles and creating the damage. This produces: 1) swelling, redness and scaling of the proximal nail fold from the mechanical injury; 2) multiple horizontal grooves that do not extend to the lateral margin of the nail—often filled with dirt, they are interspersed between the ridges; 3) a large central longitudinal or slightly lateral depression running down the nail mimicking median canaliform dystrophy, with an enlarged lunula.

Causes of transverse lines	
Common	High fever
	Post natal
	Menstrual cycle (multiple)
	Measles
	Trauma
	Chronic paronychia
	Local inflammation
	Chronic eczema
Uncommon	Kawasaki syndrome
	Stevens–Johnson syndrome
	Cytotoxic drugs
	Acrodermatitis enteropathica and zinc deficiency (Figure 2.12)
	Hypoparathyroidism
	Syphilis

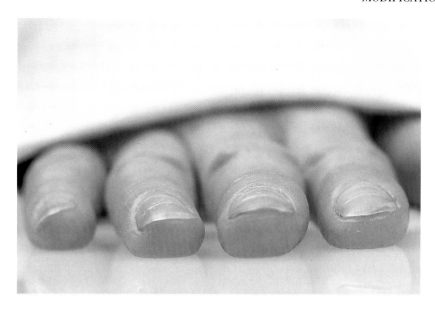

Figure 2.11 Transverse (Beau's) lines—distal view showing that lines are due to a depression.

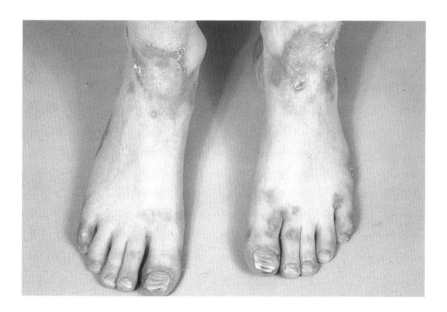

Figure 2.12 Multiple transverse nail lines in acrodermatitis enteropathica (zinc deficiency).

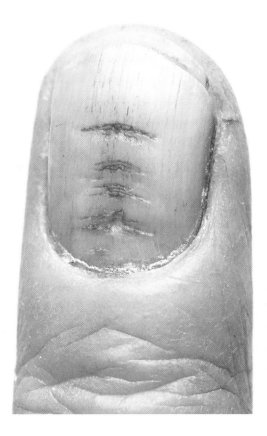

Figure 2.13 Self-inflicted multiple transverse grooves of thumb nail.

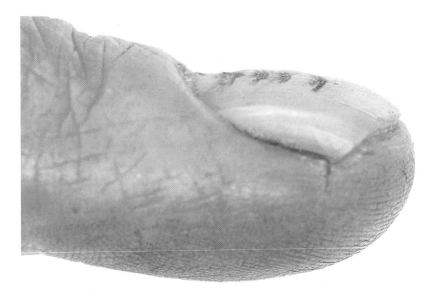

Figure 2.14 Same defect as in Figure 2.13—side view.

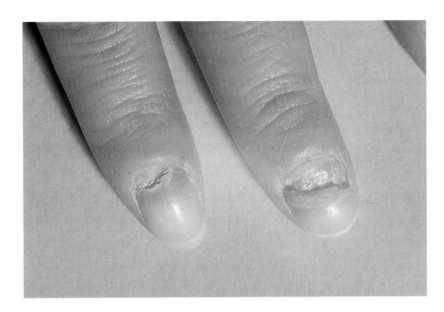

Figure 2.15   Transverse line and nail growth arrest—onychomadesis (see Chapter 3).

Pitting and rippling (Figures 2.16–2.22)

Pitting and rippling are also known as pits, onychia punctata, erosions and Rosenau's depressions (Figure 2.16–2.22).

Pits develop as a result of defective nail formation in punctate areas located in the proximal portion of the nail matrix. The surface of the nail plate is covered by small punctate depressions which vary in number, size, depth and shape. The depth and width of the pits relates to the extent of the matrix involved; their length is determined by the duration of the matrix damage.

They are randomly distributed or uniformly arranged in series along one or several longitudinal lines, or sometimes arranged in a criss-cross pattern: they may resemble the external surface of a thimble (rippled pitting).

It has been shown that regular pitting could be converted to rippling or ridging and these two conditions appear, at times, to be variants of uniform pitting (Figure 2.18). Nails showing diffuse pitting grow faster than the apparently normal nails.

Occasional pits occur on normal nails. Deep pits can be attributed to psoriasis. Shallow pits are usually seen in alopecia areata (Figure 2.21), eczema (Figure 2.22) or occupational trauma. In some cases a genetic basis is possible. In secondary syphilis and pityriasis rosea pitting occurs rarely. We have seen one case of the latter, with the pits distributed on all the finger nails at corresponding levels, in a manner analogous to Beau's lines.

The following box lists the commonest causes of nail pitting.

Causes of pitting	
Common	Psoriasis (Figure 2.16)
	Alopecia areata (Figure 2.21)
	Eczema (Figure 2.22)
	Occupational trauma
	Parakeratosis pustulosa
Uncommon	Normal
	Pityriasis rosea
	Secondary syphilis
	Sarcoid
	Reiter's syndrome
	Lichen planus

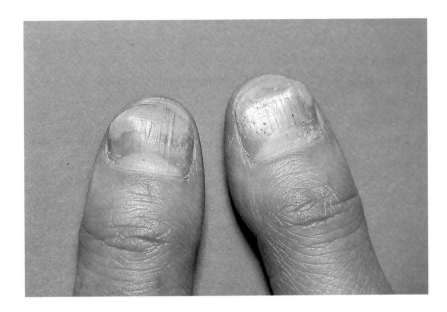

Figure 2.16   Nail pitting and onycholysis, in psoriasis.

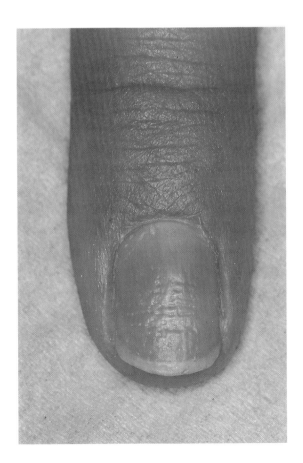

Figure 2.17   Pitting in transverse lines (regular pattern, due to alopecia areata)—see also Figure 2.18.

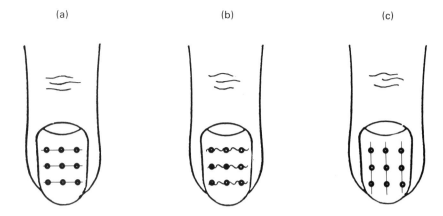

Figure 2.18   Pitting of the nail: (a) regular; (b) rippled; (c) ridged varieties.

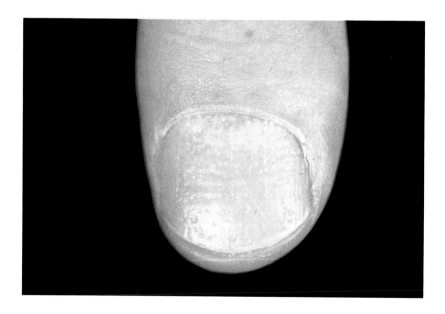

Figure 2.19   Pitting—transverse, almost rippled, pattern (see also Figure 2.18).

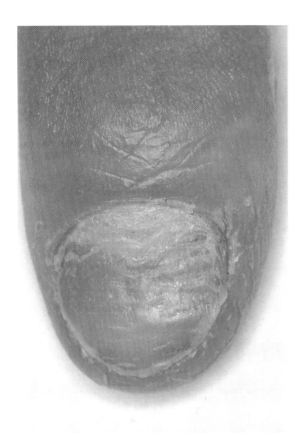

Figure 2.20 Rippled pattern of pitting—may occur as an isolated abnormality.

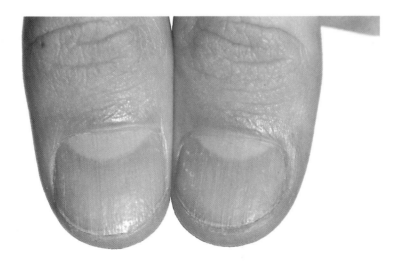

Figure 2.21 'Fine' pits in longitudinal lines, possibly due to alopecia areata.

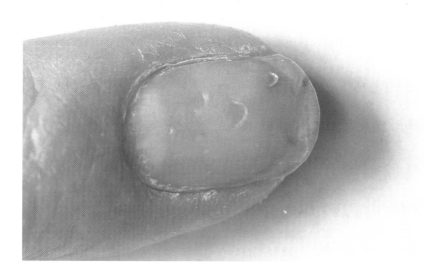

Figure 2.22   Coarse, large pits in eczema.

Trachyonychia (Rough nails) (Figures 2.23–2.26)

This sign was first used and described many decades ago in relation to congenital nail atrophies. It is characterized by a roughness of the nail surface and a grey opacity of the nail, which becomes brittle and splits at the free edge. One form may result from external chemical action; other types are idiopathic, congenital or acquired. The latter type involving all the digits may be related to a known dermatological disorder, such as lichen planus, psoriasis or alopecia areata although these conditions may not yet be manifest. Identical nail changes have been described in ichthyosis vulgaris, dark red lunulae and knuckle pads, selective IgA deficiency and ectodermal dysplasias.

'Twenty nail dystrophy of childhood' was the term coined by Hazelrigg to describe an entity already recognized as 'excess ridging' of childhood. This is an acquired, idiopathic nail dystrophy in which all twenty nails are uniformly and simultaneously affected with excess longitudinal ridging and loss of lustre (Figures 2.23, 2.24). It begins insidiously in early childhood and resolves slowly with age.

The so-called 'twenty nail dystrophy' affects both children and adults. Some clarification of the confusion in the literature regarding this condition is indicated. It can be divided into two main types:

a) The whole nail gives the appearance of having been sandpapered in a longitudinal direction. There is excessive ridging and a roughness which deprives the nail of its natural lustre. This has been designated 'vertical striated sandpaper twenty nail dystrophy'. It is most frequently associated with alopecia areata, when a specific aetiology exists. It is difficult to demonstrate the condition adequately by photography.

b) In this type of 'twenty nail dystrophy', the nail plate is shiny, with opalescent longitudinal ridging. The fine stippled aspect of the nail reflects the flash camera and is clearly evident on photography. Alopecia areata may occur in association with both types.

The pathogenesis is controversial: alopecia areata, less often lichen planus and rarely psoriasis have all been associated with the 'twenty nail dystrophy of childhood'; in one case histology revealed eczematous changes. The term has come to include such a wide variety of conditions which affect all twenty nails that it has lost its diagnostic value and should be discarded.

The following box lists the known causes and associations of this physical sign.

	Causes and associations of trachyonychia
Common	Idiopathic ('20 nail dystrophy') (Figures 2.23, 2.24)
	Alopecia areata
	Lichen planus (Figures 2.25, 2.26)
	Eczematous histology
	Chemicals
Less common	Ichthyosis vulgaris
	Ectodermal dysplasias
	Selective IgA deficiency
	Knuckle pads and dark lunulae
	Amyloidosis—systemic

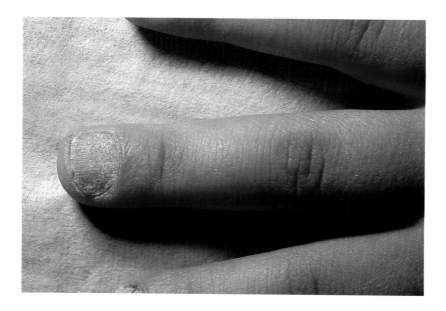

Figure 2.23   Trachyonychia in '20 nail dystrophy'.

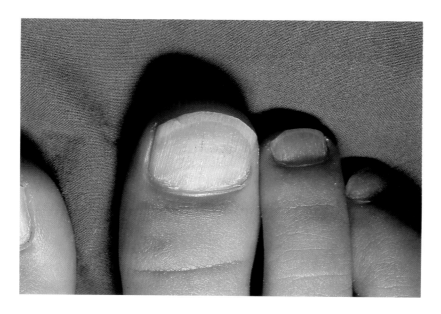

Figure 2.24   More smooth 'fine' roughness—cryptogenic '20 nail dystrophy'.

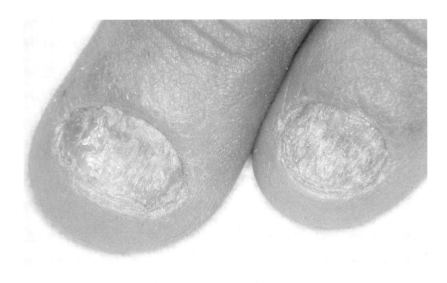

Figure 2.25   Severe trachyonychia, possibly due to lichen planus.

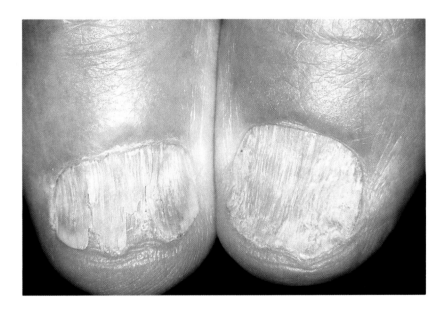

Figure 2.26   Severe lichen planus trachyonychia.

Onychoschizia (lamellar splitting) (Figures 2.27–2.34)

In this condition, the distal portion of the nail splits horizontally. The nail is formed in layers analogous to the formation of scales in the epidermis; the thin lamellae then break off. Exogenous factors contribute to the cause of the defect. It is common in housewives and others whose nails are repeatedly soaked in water, causing frequent hydration and dehydration.

Splitting into layers has been reported in X-linked dominant chondrodysplasia punctata and in polycythaemia vera. The onychoschizia may be seen in the proximal portion of the nail in lichen planus and also due to aromatic retinoid therapy.

The following box lists the known causes of onychoschizia.

Causes and lamellar splitting

Proximal	Psoriasis (Figure 2.33)
	Lichen planus
	Retinoid therapy
Distal	Chemical injury
	Old age
	Repeated nail wetting (Figures 2.30–2.32)
	Chondrodysplasia punctata—X-linked
	Polycythaemia vera

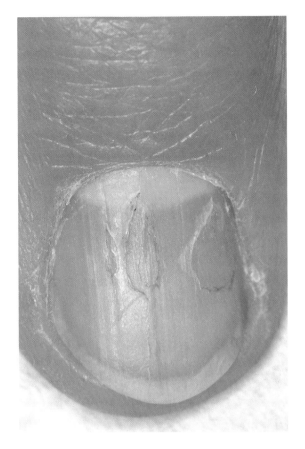

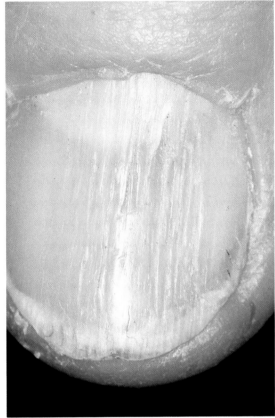

Figure 2.27   Proximal lamellar splitting due to retinoid therapy.

Figure 2.28   Longitudinal lamellar splitting.

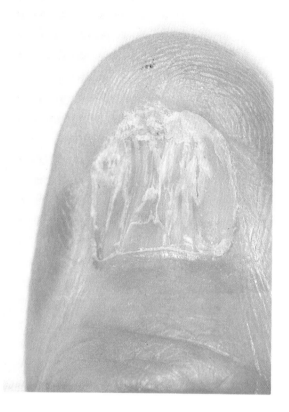

Figure 2.29   Severe superficial onychoschizia.

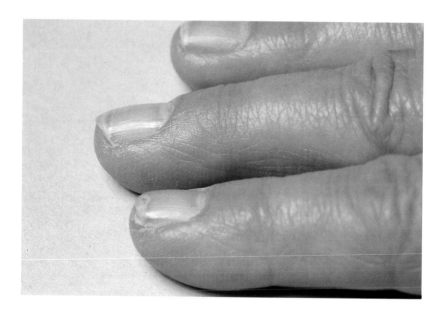

Figure 2.30   Distal lamellar splitting—often due to frequent hydration–dehydration from constant wetting.

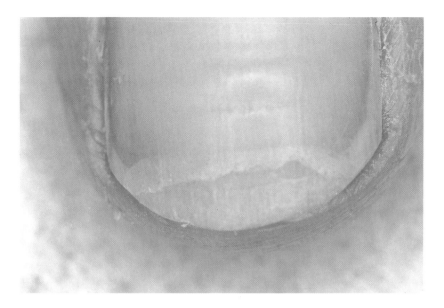

Figure 2.31   Close-up of defect seen in Figure 2.30, clearly showing the loss of nail plate in layers.

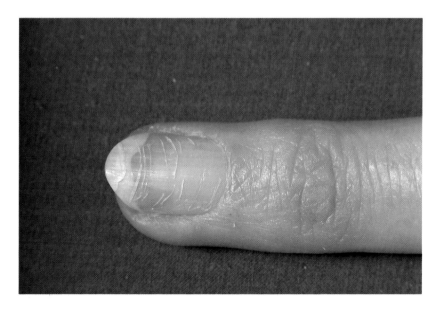

Figure 2.32   Distal and superficial lamellar splitting—constant wetting.

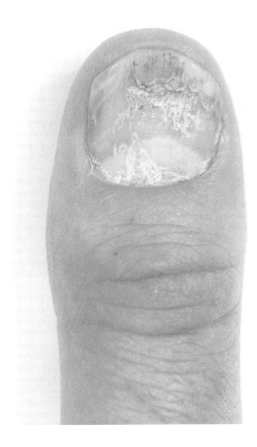

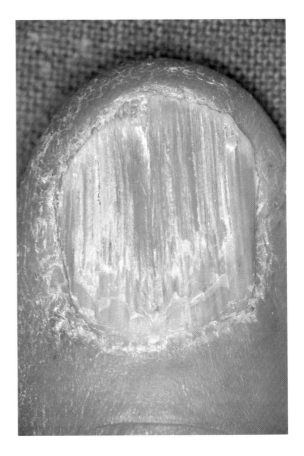

Figure 2.33 Patchy onychoschizia in psoriasis.

Figure 2.34 Severe onychoschizia and fragility (see also Chapter 5) in systemic amyloidosis.

Further reading

Trachyonychia

Baran R and **Dawber RPR,** Twenty nail dystrophy of childhood: a misnamed syndrome. *Cutis* (1987) **39**:481–2.

Onychoschizia

Shelley WB and **Shelley ED,** Onychoschizia: scanning electron microscopy. *J Am Acad Dermatol* (1984) **10**:623–7.

3

Nail plate and soft tissue abnormalities

Onycholysis (Figures 3.1–3.4)

Onycholysis refers to the detachment of the nail from its bed at its distal end and/or its lateral attachments.

The pattern of separation of the plate from the nail bed takes many forms. Sometimes it resembles closely the damage from a splinter under the nail, the detachment extending proximally along a convex line, giving the appearance of a half-moon. When the process reaches the matrix, onycholysis becomes complete. Involvement of the lateral edge of the nail plate alone is less common. In certain cases, the free edge rises up like a hood, or coils up on itself like a roll of paper. Onycholysis creates a subungual space that gathers dirt and keratinous debris; the greyish-white colour is due to the presence of air under the nail but the colour may vary from yellow to brown, depending on the aetiology. This area is sometimes malodorous.

In psoriasis there is usually a yellowish-brown margin visible between the pink, normal nail and the white, separated area. In the 'oily spot' or 'salmon-patch' variety, the nail plate–nail bed separation may start in the middle of the nail; this is sometimes surrounded by a yellow margin, especially in psoriasis. The accumulation of large amounts of serum-like exudate containing glycoprotein, in and under the affected nails, explains the colour change in this kind of onycholysis.

Glycoprotein deposition is commonly found in inflammatory and eczematous diseases affecting the nail bed. Oil patches have been reported in systemic lupus erythematosus; they may be extensive in lectitis purulenta et granulomatosa.

Onycholysis is usually symptomless and it is mainly the appearance of the nail which brings the patient to the doctor; occasionally there is slight pain associated with inflammation in the early stages. The extent of onycholysis increases progressively and can be estimated by measuring the distance separating the distal edge of the lunula from the limit of proximal detachment. Transillumination of the terminal phalanx gives a good view of the area.

The onset may be sudden, as in photo-onycholysis (Figures 3.3, 3.4) where there may be a triad of 'photosensitization, onycholysis and dyschromia'; and when the cause is contact with chemical irritants such as hydrofluoric acid. Sculptured onycholysis is a self-induced nail abnormality produced by cleaning the underside of the nail plate with a sharp instrument; this results in an opaque, distal portion of the nail with a gently curved, proximal, 'lytic' border. Sculptured onycholysis and idiopathic onycholysis of women are probably the same condition (Figure 3.1).

Onycholysis of the toe demonstrates some differences from the condition on the fingers: the major distinctions are governed by:

● the lack of occupational factors;

● the reduced use of cosmetics on the feet;

● the protection afforded by footwear which reduces the risk of photo-onycholysis.

The two main causes of onycholysis of the toe nail, especially the great toe nail, are onychomycosis and traumatic onycholysis.

Primary candida onycholysis is almost exclusively confined to the finger nails.

In distal subungual onychomycosis of the toe nails, the horny thickening raises the free edge of the nail with disruption of the normal nail plate–nail bed attachment; this gives rise to secondary onycholysis. Some authors have questioned whether great toe nail mycotic onycholysis is ever truly primary. Its presence should always lead to a search for abnormalities of the foot such as hyperkeratosis of the metatarsal heads, thickening of the ball of the foot or pressure on the big toe by an overriding second toe.

The box on page 71 lists a large number of potential causes of onycholysis. The commonest types presenting to dermatologists are due to psoriasis, onychomycosis and the cosmetic 'sculptured' varieties of adult women.

Some causes of onycholysis

Idiopathic
    Leuko-onycholysis paradentotica (Schuppli syndrome)
    Of women (probably cosmetic)

Systemic
    Circulatory (lupus erythematosus, etc)
    Yellow nail syndrome
    Endocrine (hypothyroidism, thyrotoxicosis, etc)
    Pregnancy
    Syphilis
    Iron deficiency anaemia
    Carcinoma of the lung
    Pellagra

Congenital and/or hereditary
    Partial hereditary onycholysis
    Pachyonychia congenita

Cutaneous diseases
    Psoriasis, Reiter's disease, vesiculous or bullous disease, lichen planus, alopecia areata, multicentric reticulohistiocytosis
    Atopic dermatitis, contact dermatitis (accidental or occupational), mycosis fungoides, actinic reticuloid
    Hyperhidrosis—tumours of the nail bed
    Drugs: bleomycin, doxorubicin, 5-fluoroacil, retinoids
    Drug-induced photo-onycholysis: trypaflavine, chlorpromazine, chloramphenicol, cephaloridine, cloxacillin (exceptional)
    Tetracyclines (Figure 3.3): especially demethylchlortetracycline and doxycycline but also minocycline
    Photochemotherapy with psoralens (sunlight or PUVA)
    Benoxaprofen, thiazide, diuretics, flumequine

Local causes
    Traumatic (accidental, occupational, self-inflicted or mixed) as with clawing, pinching or stabbing
    Foreign bodies
    Infectious
        Fungal
        Bacterial
        Viral (eg warts, herpes simplex, herpes zoster)
    Chemical (accidental or occupational)
    Prolonged immersion in (hot) water with alkalis and/or detergents, sodium hypochlorite etc
    Paint removers
    Sugar solution
    Gasoline and similar solvents
    Cosmetics (base coats, formaldehyde, false nails, depilatory products, nail polish removers). Nickel derived from metal pellets in nail varnish
    Physical
    Thermal injury (accidental or occupational)
    Microwaves

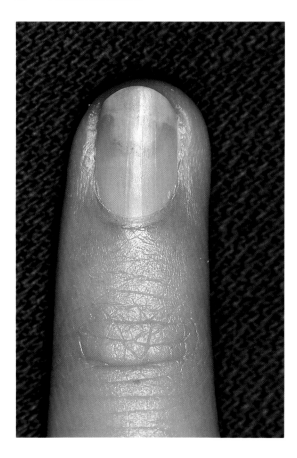

Figure 3.1   Onycholysis.

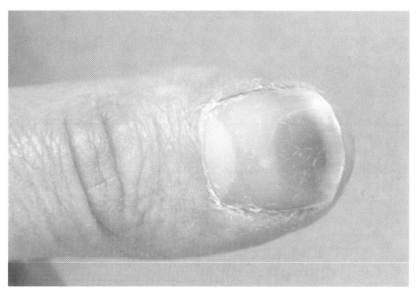

Figure 3.2   Onycholysis with green discoloration due to *Pseudomonas pyocyanea* colonization.

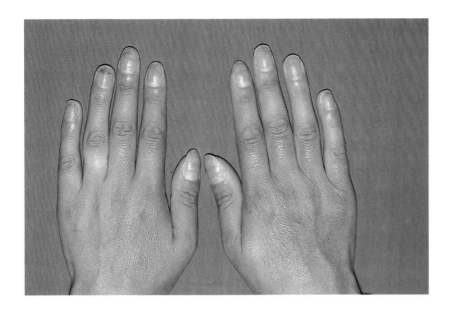

Figure 3.3 Photo-onycholysis due to oral tetracycline.

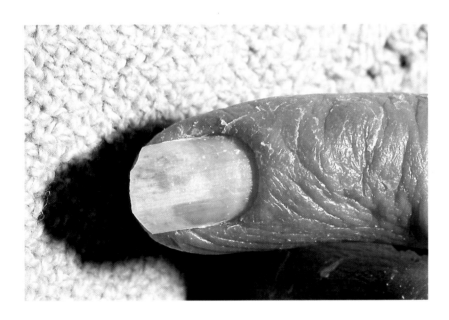

Figure 3.4 Photo-onycholysis in chronic actinic dermatitis (actinic reticuloid).

Shedding and onychomadesis (Figures 3.5–3.9)

Nails may be shed by the progression of any severe type of onycholysis causing the nail plate to separate more proximally. Onychomadesis is the spontaneous separation of the nail plate from the matrix area (Figures 3.7–3.9); this is probably associated with some arrest of nail growth—see transverse lines (Chapter 2).

At first, a cleavage appears under the proximal portion of the nail, followed by the disappearance of the juxtamatricial portion of the surface of the nail. A surface defect is thus formed, which does not usually involve the deeper layers. It is due to a limited lesion of the proximal part of the matrix.

In latent onychomadesis the nail plate shows a transverse split because of transient, complete inhibition of nail growth for at least 1 to 2 weeks. It may be characterized by a Beau's line which has reached its maximum dimensions; nevertheless the nail continues growing for some time because there is no disruption in its attachment to the underlying tissues. Growth ceases when it is cast off after losing this connection. In some, very severe, general acute diseases, such as Lyell's syndrome, the proximal edge of all the nail plates may be elevated. Growth proceeds because of the continued movement of the nail bed to which the nails remain attached.

The terms 'onychoptosis defluvium' or 'alopecia unguium' are sometimes used to describe the sign of onychomadesis. It usually results from serious generalized diseases, bullous dermatoses, drug reactions, intensive X-ray therapy, acute paronychia or severe psychological stress, or it may be idiopathic. Nail shedding may be an inherited disorder (as a dominant characteristic); the shedding may be periodic, and rarely associated with the dental condition amelogenesis imperfecta. Longitudinal fissures, recurrent onychomadesis and onychogryphosis may be associated with mild degrees of keratosis punctata. In toe nails, onychomadesis may be produced by minor traumatic episodes, as in sportsman's toe.

Total nail loss with scarring of the nail bed may be due to permanent damage of the matrix following trauma, or late stages of acquired onychatrophia following lichen planus, bullous diseases, or where there is defective peripheral circulation.

In texts on congenital anomalies, this defect is sometimes referred to as 'aplastic anonychia' which does not always produce scarring.

Temporary, total nail loss may also result from severe progressive onycholysis.

The following box lists many of the recognized causes of nail shedding.

Causes and associations of nail shedding

Local inflammation, eg acute paronychia (Figure 3.5)
Kawasaki syndrome
Fever/systemic upsets
Syphilis
Bullous dermatoses, eg pemphigus
Stevens–Johnson syndrome
Lyell's syndrome (Figure 3.7)
Drugs
  Cytotoxics
  Antibiotics
  Retinoids
Keratosis punctata
Local trauma
X-irradiation
Acrodermatitis enteropathica
Hypoparathyroidism with amelogenesis imperfecta
Yellow nail syndrome (Figure 3.6)

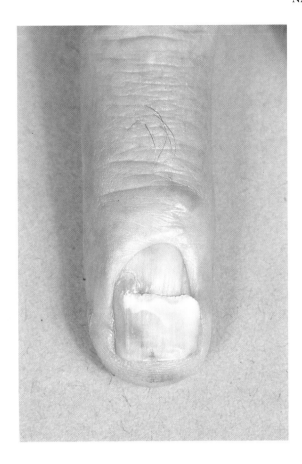

Figure 3.5 Nail shedding due to acute bacterial paronychia.

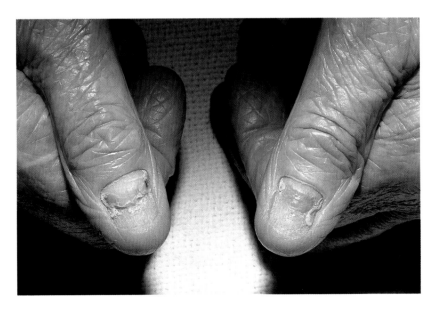

Figure 3.6 Nail shedding in yellow nail syndrome—see also Chapter 6.

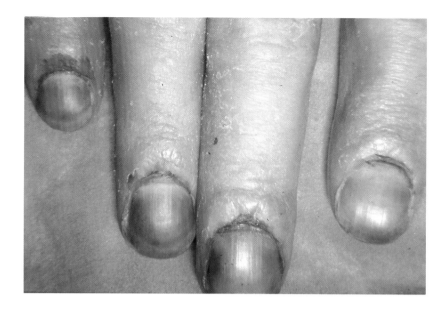

Figure 3.7   Onychomadesis in Lyell's syndrome.

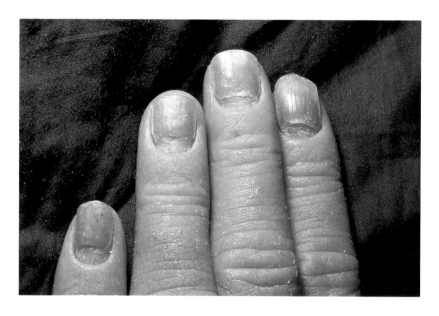

Figure 3.8   Later stage of onychomadesis than Figure 3.7.

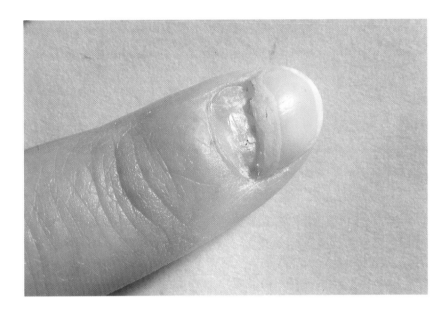

Figure 3.9 Extending onychomadesis.

Hypertrophy and subungual hyperkeratosis (Figures 3.10–3.18)

Ideally, the term 'hypertrophy of the nail plate' should be restricted to those conditions causing nail enlargement and thickening by their effects on the nail matrix (excluding nail bed and hyponychium). 'Subungual hyperkeratosis' should relate to those entities leading to thickening beneath the preformed nail plate, that is, thickening of the nail bed or hyponychial origin. In practice, this differentiation is difficult to define and 'mixed' cases are commonly seen, for example in psoriasis (Figures 3.11–3.15).

The normal thickness of fingernails is approximately 0.5 mm: this is consistently increased in manual workers and many disease states such as congenital ichthyoses, Darier's disease, psoriasis and repeated trauma. The latter particularly relates to toe nails where microtrauma and footwear are constantly affecting the nails. Onychogryphosis (Figures 3.11–3.13), a condition particularly seen in the great toe nails of elderly and infirm individuals, is probably due to trauma, footwear pressure, neglect and sometimes associated poor peripheral circulation and fungal infection; these and the less common causes are listed in the box on this page.

Epithelial hyperplasia of the subungual tissues results from exudative skin diseases and may occur with any chronic inflammatory condition which involves this area. It is especially common in psoriasis, pityriasis rubra pilaris and chronic eczema and may also be due to fungi. Histology reveals Periodic Acid Schiff reagent (PAS) positive, homogeneous rounded or oval-shaped, amorphous masses surrounded by normal squamous cells usually separated from each other by empty spaces. These clumps, which coalesce and enlarge, have also been described in alopecia areata and in some hyperkeratotic processes such as warts involving the subungual area. The horny excrescences of the nail bed are not very marked, but the ridged structure may become apparent if the nail plate is cut and shortened.

In keratosis cristarum the keratinizing process is limited to the peripheral area of the nail bed. It starts at its distal portion but may progress

somewhat proximally. Acaulis (scopulariopsis) onychomycosis may present with similar changes.

The boxes on page 79 show some examples of causes of thick nails and subungual hyperkeratosis.

Causes and associations of onychogryphosis	
Dermatological diseases	Ichthyosis Psoriasis Onychomycosis Syphilis, pemphigus, variola
Local causes (Figures 3.11–3.13)	Isolated injury to the nail apparatus Repeated minor trauma caused by footwear Foot anomalies such as hallux valgus
Regional causes	Associated varicose veins Thrombophlebitis—even in the upper limb Aneurysms Elephantiasis Pathology in the peripheral nervous system
General causes	Old age (Figures 3.11, 3.13) Tramps and senile dementia Disease involving the central nervous system
Idiopathic forms	Acquired or hereditary

Causes of thick nails
(often associated with onycholysis)

Psoriasis/Reiter's syndrome (Figures 3.11, 3.15)
Onychomycosis (Figure 3.12)
Pityriasis rubra pilaris (PRP) (Figures 3.16, 3.17)
Pachyonychia congenita (Figure 3.14)
Darier's disease (Figure 3.18)
Trauma
Contact eczema
    Mineral oils
    Cement workers
    Hair stylists
Lichen planus
Alopecia areata
Norwegian scabies
Acrokeratosis paraneoplastica (Bazex)

Causes of subungual hyperkeratosis

Chronic eczema
Darier's disease (Figure 3.18)
Distal and lateral subungual onychomycosis
Lichen planus
Norwegian scabies
Pachyonychia congenita (Figure 3.14)
Pityriasis rubra pilaris
Psoriasis
Reiter's disease

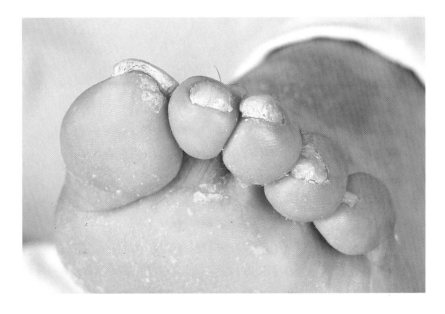

Figure 3.10   Nail plate thickening in psoriasis.

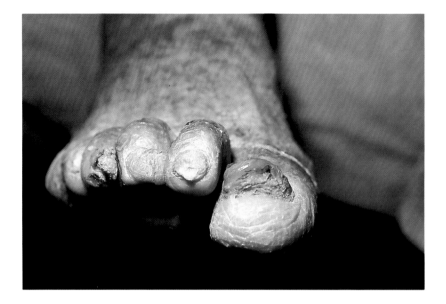

Figure 3.11   Nail plate thickening and subungual hyperkeratosis—early onychogryphosis.

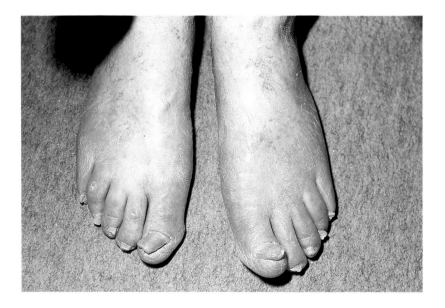

Figure 3.12   Dermatophyte nail infection with nail thickening.

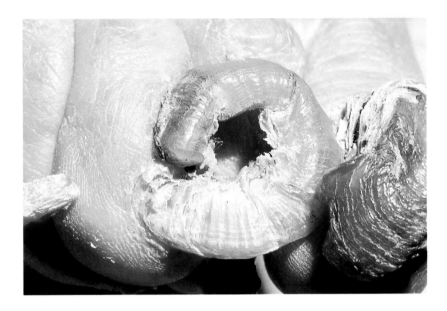

Figure 3.13 Onychogryphosis—'ram's horn' nails.

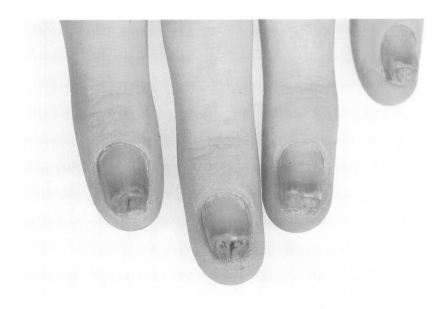

Figure 3.14 Pachyonychia congenita—nail thickening and subungual hyperkeratosis.

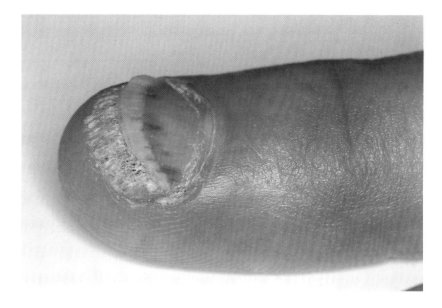

Figure 3.15   Subungual (distal) hyperkeratosis together with splinter haemorrhages—in psoriasis.

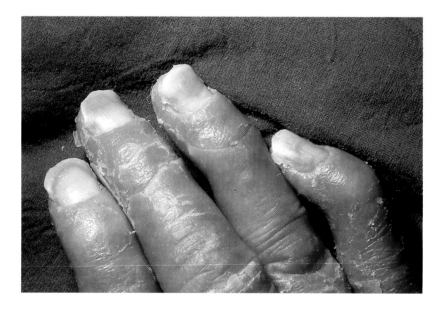

Figure 3.16   Severe pityriasis rubra pilaris with raised nails due to distal subungual thickening.

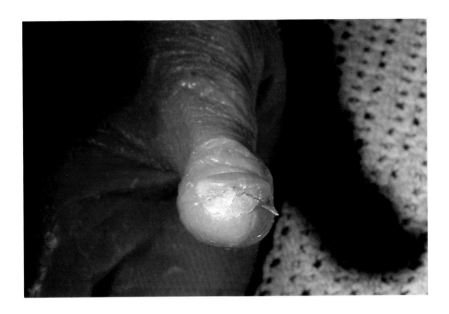

Figure 3.17   Distal view of nail seen in Figure 3.16—pityriasis rubra pilaris.

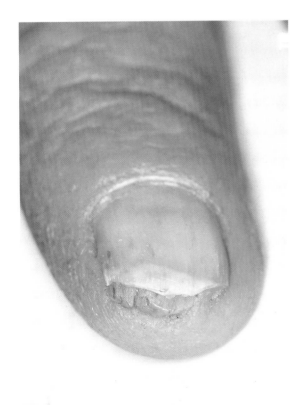

Figure 3.18   Darier's disease—distal subungual thickening.

Splinter haemorrhages and subungual haematoma (Figures 3.19–3.24)

Splinter haemorrhages (Figures 3.19–3.21)

The subungual epidermal ridges extend from the lunula distally to the hyponychium and fit 'tongue-and-groove' fashion between similarly arranged dermal ridges. The disruption of the fine capillaries along these longitudinal dermal ridges will result in splinter haemorrhages (Figure 3.19).

Macroscopically, splinter haemorrhages appear as tiny linear structures, usually not greater than 2–3 mm long, arranged in the long axis of the nail (Figures 3.20, 3.21). The majority originate within the distal one-third of the nail from the special, 'spirally wound' capillary which produces the pink line normally seen through the nail about 4 mm proximal to the tip of the finger. The whole nail bed is rarely involved by splinter haemorrhages. When first formed they are plum coloured but darken to brown or black within 1 to 2 days; subsequently they move superficially and distally with the growth of the nail, at this stage they can be scraped from the undersurface of the nail plate.

The nature of splinter haemorrhages is not clearly known. They may result from emboli in the terminal vessels of the nail bed; the emboli may be septic (Figure 3.21), or due to trauma of various types—they are commoner in the first three fingers of both hands and develop at the line of separation of the nail plate from the nail bed. Familial capillary fragility may cause splinter haemorrhages in otherwise healthy individuals. Occasional ones are of no clinical significance. There is a statistically greater incidence of splinter haemorrhages in male patients compared to females, and in Negroes compared to white individuals. In healthy females they are usually confined to a single digit. Their presence on more than one digit should raise the suspicion of an underlying pathological disorder.

Histochemical studies of nail parings confirm that the linear discoloration is derived from blood. The blood pigments give a negative Prussian blue and Pearls' reaction.

Causes of splinter haemorrhages

Arterial emboli
Arthritis (notably rheumatoid arthritis and rheumatic fever)
Behçet's disease
Blood dyscrasias (severe anaemia, high altitudes purpura)
Buerger's disease
Cirrhosis
Collagen vascular disease
Cryoglobulinaemia (with purpura)
Darier's disease
Drug reactions (especially with tetracyclines)
Eczema
Haemochromatosis
Haemodialysis and peritoneal dialysis
Heart disease (notably uncomplicated mitral stenosis and subacute bacterial endocarditis)
High-altitude living
Histiocytosis-X
Hypertension
Hypoparathyroidism
Idiopathic (probably traumatic)—up to 20 per cent of normal population
Indwelling brachial artery cannula
Malignant neoplasia
Occupational hazards
Onychomycosis
Peptic ulcer
Psoriasis
Pterygium
Pulmonary disease
Radial artery puncture
Raynaud's disease
Renal disease
Sarcoidosis
Scurvy
Septicaemia
Severe illness
Thyrotoxicosis
Trauma
Trichinosis
Vasculitis

Many conditions may be associated with the presence of splinter haemorrhages (see box). In all cases it seems probable that some aspect of the pathogenesis renders the nail bed capillaries more susceptible to minor trauma leading to linear haemorrhages.

Haematomas (Figures 3.22–3.24)

Small haemorrhages originating in the nail bed remain subungual as growth progresses distally. The deeper layers of the nail are stained by small pockets of dried blood entrapped in the nail plate. Those produced by trauma to the more proximal part of the matrix will appear in the upper layers of the plate. Sometimes patches of leukonychia are seen above haematoma.

Moderate trauma to the nail area, or blood dyscrasias, affecting extensive numbers of dermal ridges, will determine whether the haemorrhages are punctate, or result in large ecchymoses.

Acute subungual haematomas are usually obvious, occurring shortly after trauma involving finger or toe nails. The blood which accumulates beneath the nail plate produces pain which may be severe.

The size of the haematoma will determine the technique used for drainage. Treatment is required to prevent both unnecessary delay in the regrowth of the nail plate, and secondary dystrophy which might result from pressure on the matrix due to accumulated blood under the nail.

In acute haematoma of the proximal nail area, drainage of the haematoma with a fine-point scalpel blade or by drilling a hole through the plate will give prompt relief from pain. Hot paper clip cautery is a useful alternative to trephining the plate. This allows blood to be evacuated; the nail is then pressed against the bed by a moderately tight bandage, helping the nail plate to adhere. This gives good results. If this procedure is not immediately practicable, the pain can be relieved by elevating the hand as high as possible and maintaining this position for approximately 30 minutes.

Occasionally a subungual haematoma persists under the nail and does not migrate. A reddish-blue colour, an irregular shape, and an absence of colour in the nail plate help to differentiate non-migrating subungual haematomas from naevi and other causes of nail pigmentation. It is advisable to remove the part overlying the subungual haematoma and identify and remove the old dried blood in order to establish the diagnosis and to exclude more significant pathology such as malignant melanoma.

In total haematoma, often observed when there is injury to the nail bed, the possibility of an underlying fracture must be considered: X-ray is therefore required. The nail is removed, the haematoma evacuated and the wound repaired, if necessary with precise suturing of the nail bed, using 6–0 Dexon or PDS 6–0. The plate is then cleaned, shortened, narrowed and replaced by suturing to the lateral nail folds. The stitches are removed after 10 days, and usually the nail remains firmly attached.

Subungual bleeding may be due to many systemic conditions; the following box shows the morphological types most commonly seen.

Splinter haemorrhages and subungual haematoma in some systemic conditions

	Haematoma	Splinters
Arterial lines/puncture	−	+
Bacterial endocarditis	−	+
Blood dyscrasia	+	+
Cirrhosis	−	+
Collagen vascular disease	+	+
Cryoglobulinaemia	−	+
Drugs	−	+
Dialysis	−	+
Emboli	+	+
Histiocytosis-X	−	+
Scurvy	+	+
Sepsis	−	+
Thyroid	−	+
Vasculitis	−	+

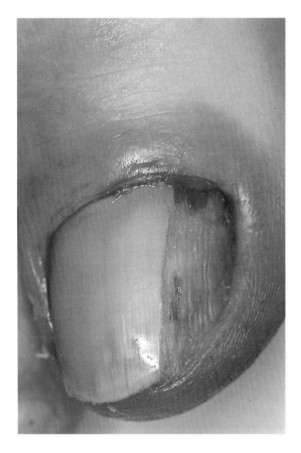

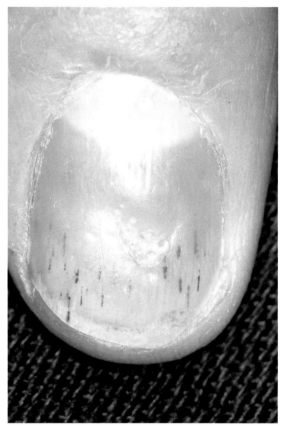

Figure 3.19 Longitudinal grooves of nail bed—the anatomical reason for linear splinter haemorrhage.

Figure 3.20 Splinter haemorrhages.

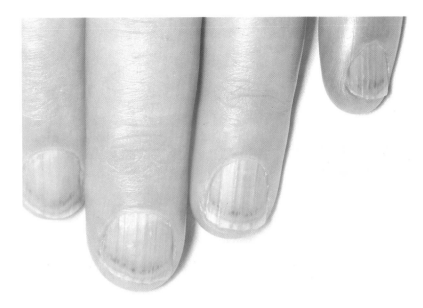

Figure 3.21   Splinter haemorrhages—microemboli from infected valvular heart disease.

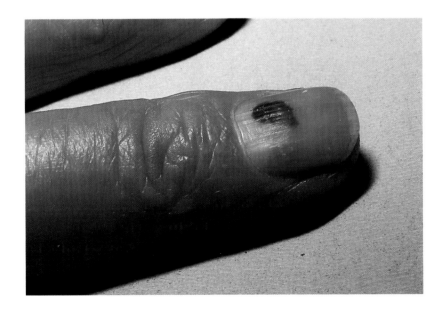

Figure 3.22   Subungual haematoma—traumatic.

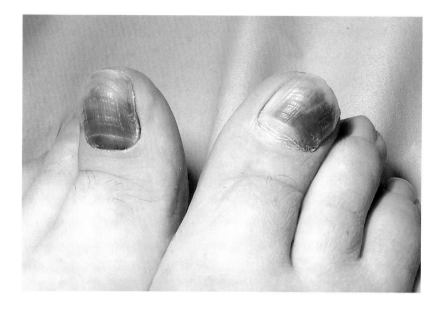

Figure 3.23   Traumatic subungual haematoma of great toe nails in a marathon runner.

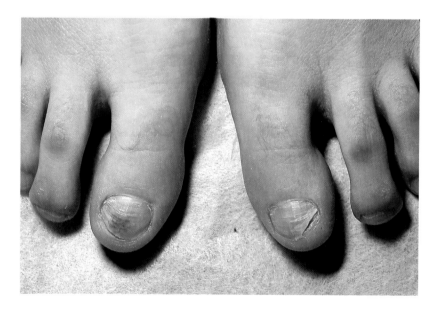

Figure 3.24   An athlete with subungual haemorrhage and onychomycosis.

Dorsal and ventral pterygium (Figures 3.25–3.29)

Dorsal pterygium consists of a gradual thinning of the proximal nail fold with associated extension of the cuticle over the nail plate (Figures 3.25–3.27). The nail plate becomes fissured because of the fusion of the cuticle to the matrix and subsequently to the nail bed; its split portions progressively decrease in size as the pterygium widens. This often results in two small nail remnants if the pterygium process is central. Complete involvement of the matrix and nail bed in the pathological process leads to total loss of the nail plate, with permanent atrophy and sometimes scarring in the nail area (see onychatrophy, page 37). Dorsal pterygium is characteristic of lichen planus and, less often, of peripheral vascular ischaemia. It also occurs in severe bullous dermatoses, radiotherapy and on the hands of radiologists: it may follow injury; rarely congenital forms have been described.

Ventral pterygium, or pterygium inversum unguis (Figures 3.28, 3.29), is a distal extension of the hyponychial tissue which anchors to the under surface of the nail, thereby eliminating the distal groove. Scarring in the vicinity of the distal groove, causing it to be obliterated, may produce secondary pterygium inversum unguis. Ventral pterygium may be seen in scleroderma associated with Raynaud's phenomenon (Figure 3.29), disseminated lupus erythematosus, and causalgia of the median nerve. The condition may be idiopathic, congenital, and familial or acquired. A congenital, aberrant, painful hyponychium has been described associated with oblique, deep fractures of the nails. There are recent reports of familial forms of the disease. In one case an unusual acquired association of pterygium inversum unguis and lenticular atrophy of the palmar creases was recorded.

Pain in the fingertip from minor trauma and haemorrhages may appear when the distal, subungual area is repeatedly pushed back or the nail cut short. Toe nails are only rarely involved.

Subungual pterygium (non-inflammatory) is analogous to the claw of lower primates.

In patients suffering from dorsal pterygium (excluding the traumatic or congenital types) the

Causes of pterygium	
Dorsal	Congenital
	Bullous dermatoses (eg cicatricial pemphigoid)
	Burns
	Dyskeratosis congenita
	Graft versus host disease
	Lichen planus (commonest cause)
	Onychotillomania
	Radiodermatitis
	Raynaud's disease and peripheral vascular disease
Ventral	Congenital
	Familial
	Idiopathic
	Peripheral neuropathy
	Raynaud's disease and systemic sclerosis
	Trauma

main characteristic is a dilatation in the nail fold capillary loops and the formation of a slender microvascular shunt system in the more dilated loops. These changes are visible using capillaroscopy.

The box above lists the well-recognized causes of pterygium. Lichen planus is the commonest specific cause of dorsal pterygium (Figures 3.25, 3.26). Ventral pterygium is most frequently seen in association with Raynaud's disease and systemic sclerosis (Figures 3.28, 3.29).

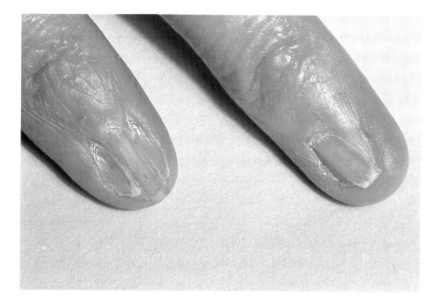

Figure 3.25   Dorsal pterygium—due to lichen planus.

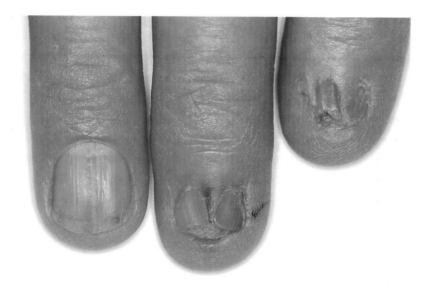

Figure 3.26   Lichen planus—severe scarring and pterygium formation.

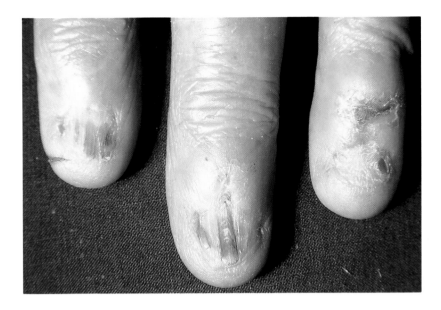

Figure 3.27   Cicatricial pemphigus showing pterygium formation.

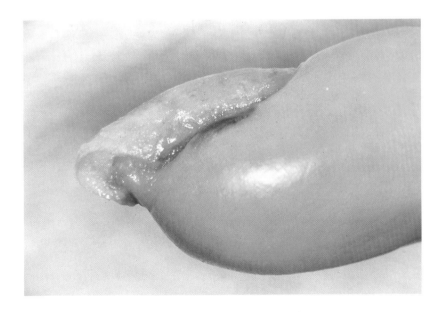

Figure 3.28   Ventral (inverse) pterygium.

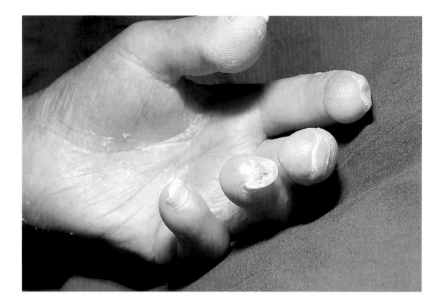

Figure 3.29   Severe acrosclerosis with painful inverse pterygium.

Further reading

Onycholysis

Kechijian P, Onycholysis of the fingernails: evaluation and management. *J Am Acad Dermatol* (1985) **12**:552–60.

Nail plate hypertrophy and subungual hyperkeratosis

DePaoli RT and **Marks VJ**, Crusted (Norwegian) scabies: treatment of nail involvement. *J Am Acad Dermatol* (1987) **17**:136–8.

Sonnex TS, Dawber RPR, Zachary CB et al, The nails in type I pityriasis rubra pilaris: a comparison with sezary syndrome and psoriasis. *J Am Acad Dermatol* (1986) **15**:956–60.

4
Periungual tissue disorders

Paronychia (Figures 4.1–4.10)

The proximal nail fold (PNF), with its distal cuticle attached to the nail and the ventral eponychium, is normally well adapted to prevent infections and external inflammatory agents entering the proximal matrix area; the same is true of the lateral nail walls and folds. It is therefore probable that no paronychia is truly primary—there always being some physical or chemical damage preceding the infection or inflammation; this is less true in relation to superficial infections on the dorsum of the PNF.

Acute paronychia (Figures 4.1, 4.2)

Minor trauma is a frequent cause of this infection and surgical treatment may be necessary. Acute paronychia may follow a break in the skin (for example, if a hang nail is torn), a splinter under the distal edge of the nail, a prick from a thorn in a lateral groove or, sometimes, from subungual infection secondary to haematoma.

The infection starts in the paronychium at the side of the nail with local redness, swelling and pain. At this stage medical treatment is indicated: wet compresses (for example with Burrow's solution) and appropriate systemic antibiotic therapy are given. Because the continuation of antibiotics may mask developing pathology which can damage the nail apparatus, if acute paronychia

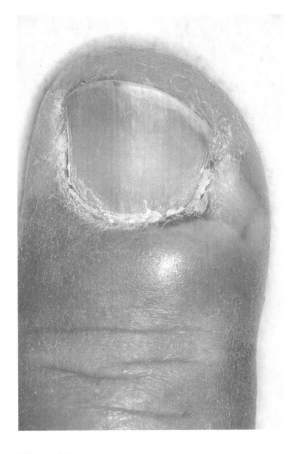

Figure 4.1 Acute bacterial paronychia.

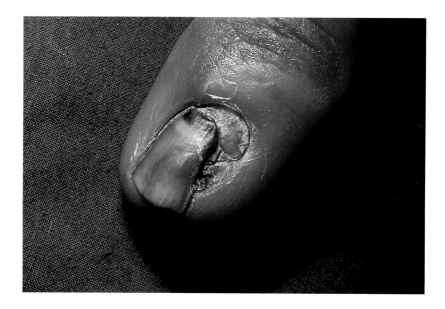

Figure 4.2   Healing stage of severe acute bacterial paronychia.

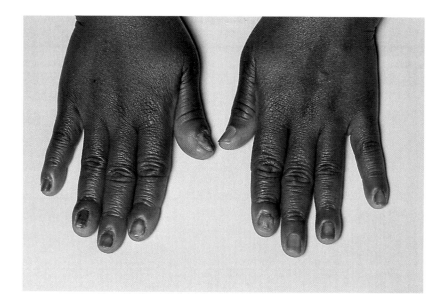

Figure 4.3   Chronic paronychia—main organism *Candida albicans*, in a domestic worker—constant wetting.

does not show clear signs of response within two days then surgical treatment should be instituted using proximal block local anaesthesia. Localization of the purulent reaction may take several days and during this time throbbing pain is always a major symptom. The collection of pus may easily be seen through the nail or at the paronychial fold. Sometimes a bead of pus may present in the periungual groove. In the absence of visible pus, the gathering gives rise to tension and the lesion should be incised at the site of maximum pain—not necessarily at the site of maximum swelling. In practice, Bunell's technique is usually successful: the base of the nail (the proximal third) is removed by cutting across with pointed scissors. A non-adherent gauze wick is laid under the proximal nail fold. If the infection in the paronychium remains restricted to one side, removal of the homologous lateral part of the nail is sufficient. Bacterial culture and sensitivity studies are of paramount importance. The bacteria most commonly found in acute paronychia are staphylococci and, less commonly, beta-haemolytic streptococci and gram-negative enteric bacteria. Should surgical intervention be delayed, the pus will track around the base of the nail under the proximal nail fold and inflame the matrix; it may then be responsible for transient or permanent dystrophy of the nail plate. It is essential to note that the nail matrix in early childhood is particularly fragile and can be destroyed within 48 hours by acute bacterial infection. The pus may also proximally separate the nail from its loose, underlying attachment. The firmer attachment of the nail at the distal border of the lunula may offer some temporary resistance to the spread of the pus. In cases of extension under part of the distal nail bed, the whole of the nail base is removed and enough nail removed distally to fully expose the involved nail bed.

Distal subungual pyogenic infection may or may not be secondary to the periungual varieties. A U-shaped piece of the distal nail plate is excised in the region loosened by the pus and debridement of the affected nail bed carried out. Extension of the infection may involve the finger pulp or the matrix.

Sometimes the evacuation of a perionychial phylctenular abscess brings to light a narrow sinus; this may be part of a 'collar-stud' abscess which communicates with a deeper, necrotic zone; it must be exposed and excised.

If acute paronychia accompanies ingrowing nail, the treatment must be supplemented by removing all offending portions of the nail plate. After surgery, the dressing is kept moist with saline or an antiseptic soak. This should be changed every day after a bath with antiseptic soap until the discharge of pus stops, with full splinting and immobilization of finger, hand and forearm, if possible.

In acute paronychia it is common for only one nail to be involved. In chronic or subacute paronychia, which may mimic acute paronychia, one or several finger nails may be infected. The differential diagnosis includes:

● paronychial involvement of the finger nails accompanying chronic eczema

● psoriasis and Reiter's disease, which may also involve the proximal nail fold.

Chronic paronychia (Figures 4.3–4.7)

Hands which are repeatedly traumatized by immersion in water become vulnerable to chronic mycotic paronychia. The condition is prevalent in people in contact with water, soap, detergents and other chemicals, particularly housewives. There is also a high incidence among chefs, barmen, confectioners and fishmongers. Paronychia may also develop in patients with skin disease such as eczema or psoriasis involving the nail folds. The index and middle fingers of the right hand and the middle finger of the left hand are most often affected; these are the digits which are most subject to minor trauma, such as rubbing during hand-washing of clothes. The onset of infection is usually insidious. It starts with erythema and swelling, often in the vicinity of a lateral nail fold with loss of the adjacent cuticle. The lesion is usually tender. After several months or even years

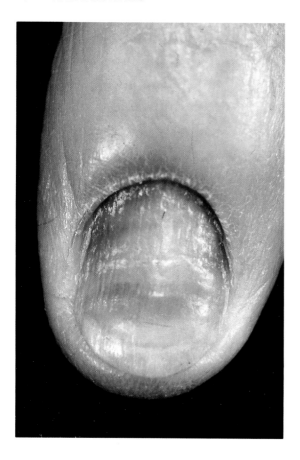

Figure 4.4   Chronic paronychia with associated nail dystrophy.

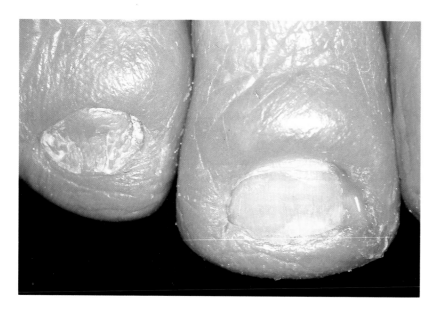

Figure 4.5   Paronychia due to etretinate therapy.

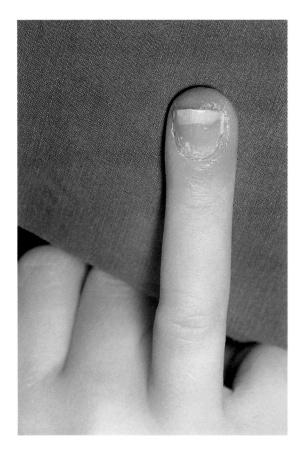

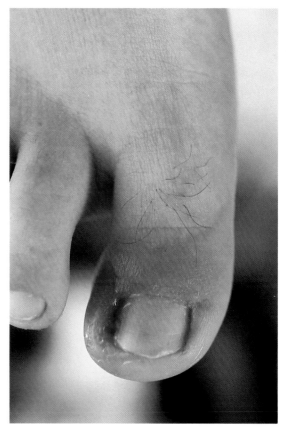

Figure 4.6 Paronychia due to finger sucking (monilial infection).

Figure 4.7 Ingrowing toe nail with lateral wall, nail fold infection.

the perionychial tissue comes to resemble a semicircular indurated cushion around the base of the nail plate, and it retracts and separates from the latter. Often a small bead of pus may be expressed from one corner of the nail fold for microscopy and culture. This procedure is sometimes painful. The pus is formed within the pocket under the fold, and is not the product of an

abcess within the perionychium. From time to time the persistent low-grade inflammation may be subject to subacute painful exacerbations which cause disturbance of the growth of the nail plate and a change in its colour, contour and surface. In the early stages the nail plate is unaffected, but one or both lateral edges may develop irregularities and yellow, brown or

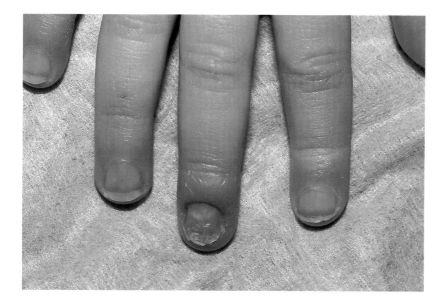

Figure 4.8   Paronychial inflammation in parakeratosis pustulosa—9-year-old girl.

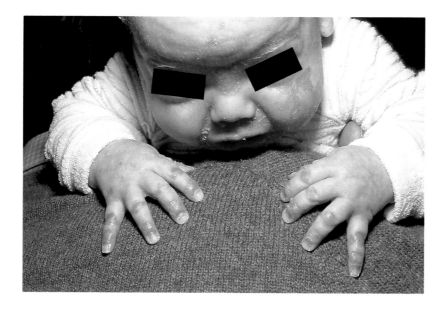

Figure 4.9   Acrodermatitis enteropathica (zinc deficiency) with paronychia inflammation—may be painful.

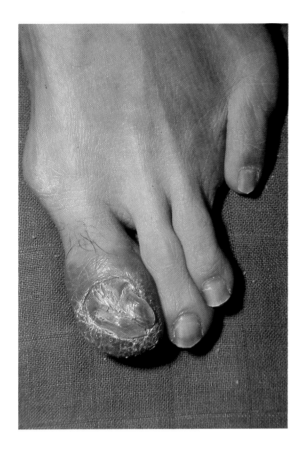

Figure 4.10 Paronychia and nail dystrophy due to sarcoidosis of the terminal phalanx (courtesy of Prof G Moulin, Lyon).

blackish discoloration; this may subsequently extend over a large portion of the nail and occasionally the whole nail becomes involved. It is believed to follow discoloration caused by dihydroxyacetone produced by the organisms in the nail fold. By contrast *Pseudomonas* often produces a greenish discoloration. The lateral discoloured edges of the nail plate become cross-ridged when the disease is predominantly confined to the lateral nail fold. On the surface, which often becomes rough and friable, numerous irregular transverse ridges or waves appear as a result of

subsequent repeated acute exacerbations. After a time the size of the nail is considerably reduced, an effect which is exaggerated by the swelling of the surrounding soft tissues.

After the paronychium has been treated successfully the onychia normally regresses, but sometimes it persists or may even continue to increase. It is then difficult to distinguish between onychia caused by pyogenic bacteria or *Candida*. There is some disagreement as to the importance of the yeast in chronic *Candida* paronychia. The various factors which damage the area allow

Staphylococcus aureus and *Candida* species to attack the keratin and cause the detachment of the cuticle from the nail plate. But *Candida* species may also act by simple colonization of the pocket under the proximal nail fold. Many authorities believe that chronic paronychia is usually a mixed infection of *C albicans* and intestinal bacteria (Streptococci, coliforms, *Proteus* and *Pseudomonas* species).

Acute exacerbations are usually caused by secondary bacterial infection and may subside without treatment. *Candida* paronychia is frequently prolonged despite treatment. The organism may be derived from the mouth and the bowel (not usually the vagina) of the patient or family members, who may be sources of *C albicans* or foreign material, including debris derived from the infective process. Persistence may also be due to continued exposure to predisposing conditions such as frequent immersion of hands in water. The reaction in the dermis produces a rounding off of the proximal nail fold, a response which tends to entrap debris and organisms, leading to chronicity of the condition. Foreign material such as wax, hair and foodstuffs may collect in the proximal nail fold. This may cause retraction of the nail fold and persistence of the process. The development of immediate or delayed type hypersensitivity to chemicals contained in food items may contribute to the pathogenesis of chronic paronychia and even be the main factor.

In children the most common predisposing factor to *Candida* paronychia is the habit of thumb- or finger-sucking. This is potentially more harmful than occupational immersion as saliva is more irritating than water (Figure 4.6).

Although infrequent, chronic paronychia of the toe nails may develop in association with diabetes mellitus or peripheral vascular disease, both of which should be excluded unless ingrowing nail is present.

Differential diagnosis

Chronic paronychia may be associated with nail infections caused by *Hendersonula toruloidea* or *Scytalidium hyalinum*. Brown discoloration starting at the lateral edges of the nail and spreading centrally into the nail has been seen in some cases. Rarely this is caused by a separate *Candida* infection which is not directly related to the original *Hendersonula* or *Scytalidium* infection.

Causes of paronychia		
Infective	Acute	Viral
		Bacterial (Figures 4.1, 4.2)
		Fungal
		Parasitic (tungiasis)
	Chronic	Mycotic (Figures 4.3, 4.4)
		Mycobacterial
		Syphilitic
Drugs	Retinoids (Figure 4.5)	
Cosmetic	Trauma	
	Epoxy resin dermatitis	
Occupational		
Dermatoses	Acrodermatitis enteropathica (Figure 4.9)	
	Darier's disease	
	Dyskeratosis congenita	
	Eczema	
	Ingrowing toe nail (Figure 4.7)	
	Lichen planus	
	Pachyonychia congenita	
	Parakeratosis pustulosa	
	Pemphigus	
	Psoriasis Reiter	
	Radiodermatitis	
	Yellow nail	
Systemic disease	Collagen vascular diseases	
	Encephalitis	
	Frostbite	
	Histiocytosis-X	
	Leukaemia	
	Metastases	
	Neuropathy	
	Paraneoplastic acrokeratosis	
	Sarcoid	
	Stevens–Johnson syndrome	
	Vasculitis	
Miscellaneous	Finger-sucking children (Figure 4.6)	

Syphilitic paronychia is due to a chancre on the perionychial area which is usually painful.

Pemphigus of the nail bed may produce considerable bolstering of the nail fold and closely resembles chronic paronychia with accompanying onychomycosis.

Parakeratosis pustulosa (Hjorth–Sabouraud's syndrome) may also mimic fungal paronychia.

Psoriatic lesions, Reiter's disease and eczema sometimes involve the proximal nail fold. Secondary bacterial or yeast infections may develop in the area.

If chronic paronychia becomes recalcitrant and unresponsive to medical procedures, then surgical removal of the proximal nail fold and proximal lateral nail folds together with the proximal nail plate may be required—after this procedure complete healing normally takes approximately 8 weeks.

The box on page 100 shows the principal causes of paronychia. Acute paronychia is most commonly seen in nail-biters, whilst the most frequently seen type of chronic paronychia is that occurring on the hands of domestic and office cleaners and bar staff (wet work) (Figures 4.2, 4.3).

Ragged cuticles and 'hang nail' (Figures 4.11–4.15)

Thickened, hyperkeratotic, irregular (ragged) cuticles are most commonly seen in association with dermatomyositis (Figures 4.14, 4.15). Perionychial tissues are constantly subjected to trauma. In nail biters and 'pickers' the cuticles and nail folds may show considerable damage (Figure 4.13), erosions, haemorrhage and crusting. The ulnar side of the nail fold and cuticle is most vulnerable and there may be small triangular tags of skin (hang nail) and separated spicules of nail, still attached proximally (Figures 4.11, 4.12). Hang nails may also result from occupational injuries, with the hydration and dehydration caused by frequent wetting. In subjects with dry skin, particularly in winter, painful dorso-lateral fissures may be seen located distal to the lateral nail groove.

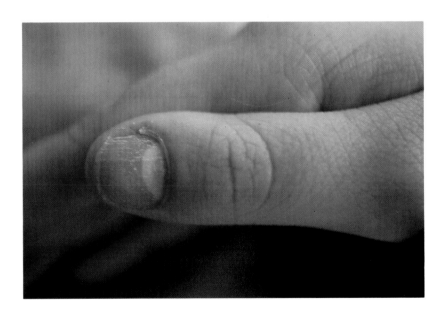

Figure 4.11   Hang nail adjacent to a thumb in a child with '20 nail dystrophy'.

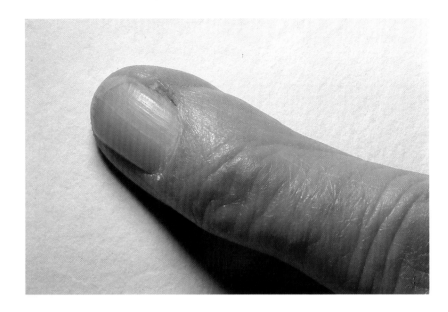

Figure 4.12 Hang nail (index finger) mimicking periungual fibroma.

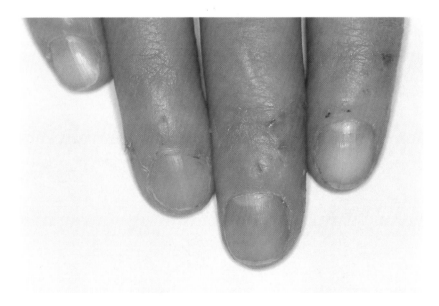

Figure 4.13 Self-induced periungual skin 'picking' and ragged cuticle—without nail biting in this case.

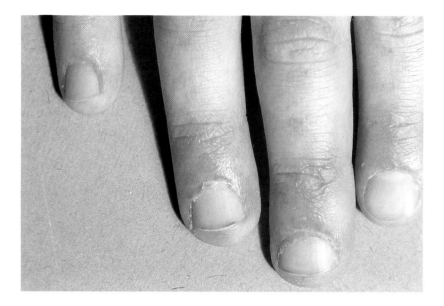

Figure 4.14 Ragged cuticles in dermatomyositis with dilated nail fold capillaries.

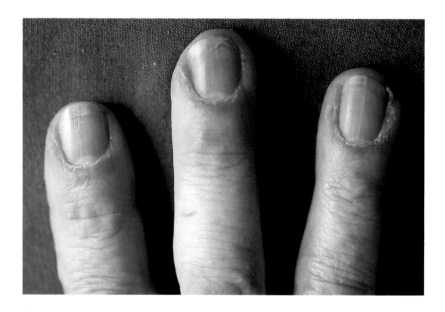

Figure 4.15 Ragged cuticles and nail fold erythema—dermatomyositis.

Tumours and swellings (Figures 4.16–4.36)

The nail apparatus develops in utero from primitive skin and it is therefore not surprising that many of the swellings and tumours that affect the rest of the skin can occur within it. The box on page 125 shows the vast array of such conditions which have been described in and around the nail apparatus; only the distinctive lesions which are peculiar to the nail apparatus and those which have different morphology in this site will be described in detail (those underlined in the box). The box on page 126 shows some of the commoner lesions related to their site within the nail apparatus.

Periungual and subungual warts (Figures 4.16–4.18)

Common warts are caused by human papilloma viruses of different biological types. They are benign, weakly contagious, fibro-epithelial tumours with a rough keratotic surface. Usually periungual warts are asymptomatic though fissuring may cause pain. Subungual warts initially affect the hyponychium, growing slowly toward the nail bed and finally elevating the nail plate. Bone erosion from verruca vulgaris occasionally occurs, though some of these cases may be

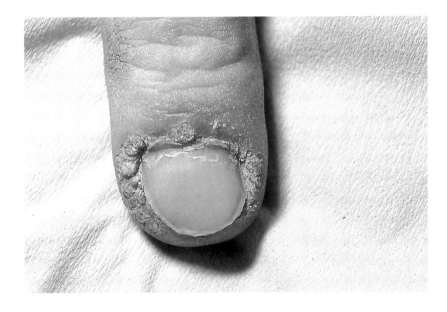

Figure 4.16   Periungual wart.

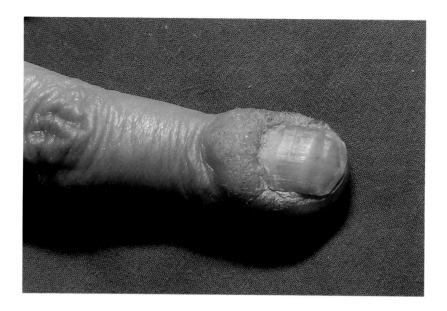

Figure 4.17   Severe periungual wart and nail dystrophy.

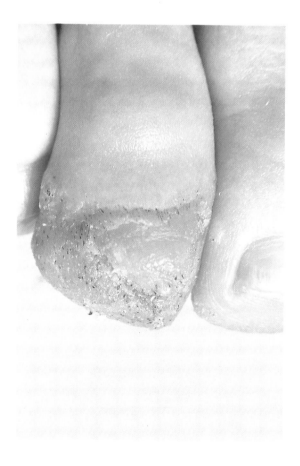

Figure 4.18   Subungual and periungual wart—fourth toe.

keratocanthomas since the latter, epidermoid carcinoma and verruca vulgaris are sometimes indistinguishable from clinical signs alone.

Subungual warts are painful and may mimic glomus tumour. The nail plate is not often affected, but surface ridging may occur and more rarely dislocation of the nail. Biting, picking and tearing of the nail and nail walls are common habits in subjects with periungual warts. This type of trauma is responsible for the spread of warts and their resistance to treatment.

Tuberculosis cutis verrucosa (butcher's nodule) may rarely pose differential diagnostic difficulties, but it is very rare in the periungual location, affecting a lateral fold of the toe nails with long-standing warty lesions with unusual wart morphology. Bowen's disease must be considered, as should the subcutaneous vegetations of systemic amyloidosis.

Treatment of periungual warts is often frustrating. X-ray and radium treatment has become obsolete. Saturated monochloroacetic acid has been suggested but is painful; it is applied sparingly, allowed to dry and then covered with 40 per cent salicylic acid plaster cut to the size of the wart and held in place with adhesive tape for 2–3 days. After 1–2 weeks many of the warts can be removed and the procedure repeated. Subungual warts are treated similarly, after cutting away the overlying part of the nail plate. Recalcitrant warts may respond to weekly applications of diphenciprone solutions ranging from 0.2 to 2 per cent according to the patient's ability to produce a good inflammatory reaction. Some authorities recommend the use of cantharidin (0.07 per cent); this is applied to the lesions and covered by a plastic tape for 24 hours. The resultant blister should be re-treated at 2-week intervals, three to four times if necessary. Recent work strongly recommends bleomycin for recalcitrant warts; it is given intralesionally $1 \mu g$ per ml at 2-week intervals. Some patients find this more painful than correctly used cryosurgery.

Surgical treatment should be avoided if possible. Cryosurgery with carbon dioxide snow or liquid nitrogen is often used but may cause blistering, with the blister roof containing the epidermal wart component if the treatment succeeds. However, when treating the proximal nail fold freezing must not be prolonged since one may easily damage the matrix; this may result in circumscribed leukonychia or even nail dystrophy, though scarring is rare with cryosurgery. Particular side-effects of cryosurgery include pain, depigmentation and secondary bacterial infection (rare); Beau's lines, onychomadesis, nail loss or inordinate oedema, the latter often worse in the very young and very old, and transient neuropathy or anaesthesia. Many of the side-effects are avoidable if the freeze times used are carefully controlled, and prophylactic analgesic and subsequent anti-inflammatory treatment is carried out—soluble aspirin 600 mg three times daily for 5 days and topical steroid application twice daily. Destruction using curettage and electrodesiccation usually produces considerable scarring. Recently infra-red coagulation and argon and carbon dioxide laser treatments have been used with some success. If the most aggressive measures fail, or compliance is poor, formalin may be applied daily with a wooden toothpick. If the lesions become inflamed, fissured or tender, because of the therapy or secondary infection, treatment is interrupted and a topical antiseptic preparation used for several days.

Many lay and medical people have 'tricks' for attempting to cure warts, such as 'wrapping' followed 2 weeks later by the careful application of liquified phenol, then a drop of nitric acid to the lesion. The fuming and spluttering that occurs looks efficaceous and the wart turns brown.

Since the incubation period of human warts may be up to several months, consistent follow-up, even after seemingly successful therapy, is necessary to allow for early treatment of newly growing warts.

Fibromas (Figures 4.19, 4.20)

There are many different types of fibromas which may develop in the subungual and periungual area. They may represent true entities in

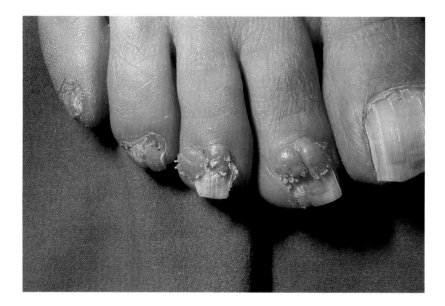

Figure 4.19   Periungual fibromas in tuberous sclerosis (Koenen's tumours).

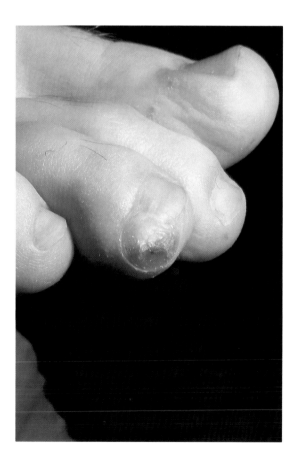

Figure 4.20   Periungual fibrokeratoma.

themselves, or merely be variants of the same process.

Keloids

Hypertrophic scars and keloids result from injuries to the nail fold or nail bed and may produce disturbances in the nail unit.

Fibromas

True fibromas are rare. They may resemble cutaneous horns, fibrokeratomas or supernumerary digits; the latter, however, usually arise on the ulnar aspect of the fifth metacarpophalangeal joint. Histologically, they are composed of very dense connective tissue bundles with elastic fibres and are sharply delineated from the normal dermal connective tissue.

Koenen's tumour (Figure 4.19)

Koenen's periungual fibromas develop in 50 per cent of the cases of tuberous sclerosis (epiloia or Bourneville–Pringle disease). They usually appear between the ages of 12 and 14 years and increase progressively in size and number with age. Individual tumours are small, round, flesh-coloured and asymptomatic, with a smooth surface.

The tip may be slightly hyperkeratotic, resembling fibrokeratoma. They grow out of the nail fold, eventually overgrowing the nail bed and destroying the nail plate. Depending on their location, they may cause longitudinal depressions in the nail plate. Excessively large tumours are often painful and should be excised at their base.

Histological changes consist of dense angio-fibrotic tissue, sometimes with neuroglial tissue at the centre, and hyperkeratosis at the tip.

Koenen's tumours are cured by simple excision. Usually no suture is necessary. Tumours growing out from under the proximal nail fold are removed after reflecting the proximal nail fold back by making lateral incisions down each margin in the axis of the lateral nail grooves. Subungual fibromas are removed after avulsion of the corresponding part of the nail plate.

Acquired periungual fibrokeratoma (Figure 4.20)

Acquired periungual fibrokeratomas are probably identical to acquired digital fibrokeratomas and Steel's garlic clove fibroma. They are acquired, benign, spontaneously developing, asymptomatic nodules with a hyperkeratotic tip and a narrow base which occur mostly in the periungual area or elsewhere on the fingers. A case was described in which the lesion was located beneath the nail and visible under the free margin of the great toe nail. Most periungual fibrokeratomas emerge from the most proximal part of the nail sulcus growing on the nail and causing a sharp longitudinal depression. Trauma is thought to be a major factor initiating acquired periungual fibrokeratoma.

Microscopically, acquired periungual fibrokeratomas resemble hyperkeratotic 'dermal herniae'. The core consists of mature eosinophilic collagen fibres orientated along the main vertical axis of the tumour. The connective tissue cells are increased. Most fibromas are highly vascular. The epidermis is thick and acanthotic. There is a marked orthokeratotic horny layer, which sometimes is parakeratotic and contains serum or blood at the tip of the tumour. Elastic fibres are normal. Acid mucopolysaccharides are not increased.

Surgical treatment is the same as for Koenen's tumours and will depend on the size and location of the fibromas.

The differential diagnosis of acquired periungual fibroma includes fibroma, keloid, Koenen's tumour, recurring digital fibrous tumours of childhood, dermatofibrosarcoma, fibrosarcoma, acrochordon, cutaneous horn, eccrine poroma, pyogenic granuloma, verruca vulgaris and exostosis.

Subungual filamentous tumour

Subungual filamentous tumours are thread-like, horny, subungual lesions growing with the nail plate and emerging from under the free edge of it. They may cause a longitudinal rim. This entity is probably a narrow, extremely hyperkeratotic fibrokeratoma; it pares down painlessly when the nail is cut.

Recurring digital fibrous tumours of childhood
(Benign juvenile digital fibromatosis)

Recurring digital fibrous tumours (RDFT) are round, smooth, firm tumours with a reddish or livid-red colour, which are located on the dorsal and axial surfaces of the fingers and toes, characteristically sparing the thumbs and great toes. They may present at birth or develop during infancy, though one single case was recently described in an adult. There is no sex predominance. Fingers are more often affected than toes. On reaching the nail unit, they may elevate the nail plate leading to dystrophy but not to destruction. Often the tumour is multicentric occurring on several digits. Although an infectious origin is probable, no virus has been isolated and viral particles have not been demonstrated by electron microscopy. Recurrence occurs in 60 per cent after excision. Spontaneous regression was noted in 5 of 61 cases; regression may be hastened by cryosurgery; however, excessive growth was treated by amputation of the involved digit in some cases. Radical surgical ablation of the area involved may be necessary, including the nail unit, leading to premanent loss of the nail. Firm plantar nodules may be associated with these tumours.

Histology shows a diffuse proliferative cellular process in the dermis with increased numbers of normal-looking fibroblasts with uniform spindle-shaped nuclei. Mitoses are absent or rare. Elastic tissue is decreased. In about 2 per cent of the fibroblasts, paranuclear inclusion bodies, 3 to 10 μm in diameter, can be seen in properly fixed specimens using stains such as iron haematoxylin,

methyl green-pyronin, and phosphotungstic acid-haematoxylin. Electron microscopy shows that the inclusions consist of fibrillar masses without a limiting membrane. On the basis of this evidence, it has been suggested that the condition should be termed 'elastodysplasia'.

Glomus tumour (Figure 4.21)

The glomus tumour was first described almost 200 years ago as a painful subcutaneous 'tubercle'.

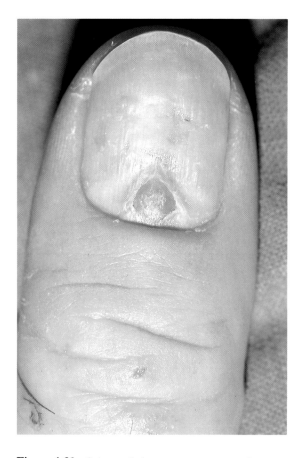

Figure 4.21   Subungual glomus tumour—exposed.

Several cases were described as malignant angiosarcomas or colloid sarcomas.

Seventy-five per cent of glomus tumours occur in the hand, especially in the fingertips and particularly the subungual area. 1–2 per cent of all hand tumours are glomus tumours. The average age of the patings at the time of diagnosis ranges from 30 to 50 years. Men are less frequently affected than women.

The glomus tumour is characterized by intense, often pulsating pain that may be spontaneous or provoked by the slightest trauma. Even changes in temperature, especially from warm to cold, may trigger pain radiating up to the shoulder. Sometimes the pain is worse at night: it may disappear when a tourniquet is applied.

The tumour is seen through the nail plate as a small, bluish to reddish-blue spot several millimetres in diameter, rarely exceeding 1 cm in diameter. Sometimes it causes a slight rise in surface temperature; this can be detected by thermography. One-half of the tumours cause minor nail deformities, ridging or a nail plate 'gutter' being the commonest. About 50 per cent cause a depression on the dorsal aspect of the distal phalangeal bone or even a cyst visible on X-ray. Probing and transillumination may help to localize the tumour if it is not clearly visible through the nail. If the tumour cannot be localized clinically or on X-ray, arteriography should be performed; this will reveal a star-shaped telangiectatic zone.

Many patients give a history of trauma. The most common misdiagnoses are neuroma, causalgia, gout, and arthritis.

Histology shows a highly differentiated, organoid tumour. It consists of an afferent arteriole, vascular channels lined with endothelium and surrounded by irregularly arranged cuboidal cells with round dark nuclei and pale cytoplasm. Primary collecting veins drain into the cutaneous veins. Myelinated and non-myelinated nerves are found and may account for the pain. The tumour is surrounded by a fibrous capsule. Since all the elements of the normal globus are present, the glomus tumour may be considered more a hamartoma than a true tumour.

The only treatment is surgical removal. Small tumours may be removed by punching a 6 mm hole in the nail plate, incising the nail bed and enucleating the lesion. The small nail disc is put back in its original position as a physiological dressing. Larger tumours may be treated after removal of the proximal half of the nail plate; thoses in lateral positions are removed by an L-shaped incision parallel to and 4–6 mm on the volar side of the lateral nail fold. The nail bed is carefully dissected from the bone until the tumour is reached and extirpated. Extirpation is usually curative, although the pain may take several weeks to disappear. Recurrences occur in 10 to 20 per cent of cases and may represent either incomplete excision or tumours overlooked at the initial operation; or newly developed tumours. More extensive surgery than is often carried out might achieve more first-time cures.

Subungual exostosis (Figures 4.22–4.24)

Subungual exostoses are not true tumours but rather outgrowths of normal bone or calcified cartilaginous remains. Whether or not subungual osteochondroma is a different entity is not clear.

Subungual exostoses are painful osseous growths which elevate the nail. They are particularly frequent in young people and are mostly located in the great toe, though subungual exostoses may also occur in the fingers. They start as small elevations of the dorsal aspect of the distal phalanx and may eventually emerge from under the nail edge or destroy the nail plate. If the nail is lost, the surface becomes eroded and secondarily infected, sometimes mimicking an ingrown toe nail. Walking may be painful.

Trauma appears to be a major causative factor, though some authors claim that a history of trauma is only occasionally found in subungual exostosis.

The triad of pain (the leading symptom), nail deformation, and radiographic features is usually diagnostic. The exostosis is a trabeculated osseous growth with an expanded distal portion covered with radiolucent fibrocartilage.

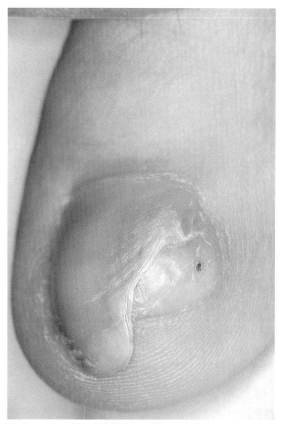

(a) (Courtesy of Prof E Haneke, Wuppertal.)

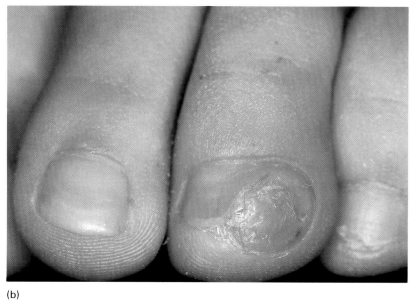

(b)

Figure 4.22   Subungual exostosis.

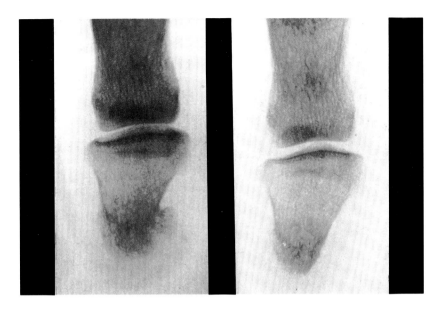

Figure 4.23 Subungual exostosis—same condition as Figure 4.22, two X-ray views.

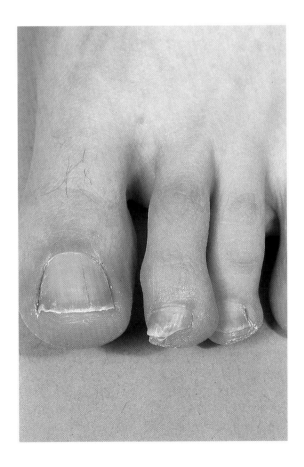

Figure 4.24 Subungual exostosis on the second toe—similar appearance to subungual wart.

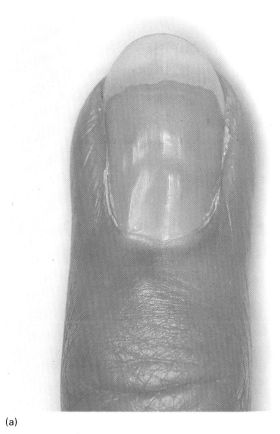

(a)

(b)

Figure 4.25 Atypical myxoid cysts: (a) myxoid cyst superficial to the nail matrix produces a groove in the nail plate; (b) myxoid cyst under the nail matrix producing filing and flaking of the nail plate.

Osteochondroma, commonly evoking the same symptoms, is said to have a male predominance. There is often a history of trauma. Its growth rate is slow. X-ray shows a well-defined sessile bone growth with a hyaline cartilage cap which must be differentiated from primary subungual calcification, particularly seen in older women, and secondary subungual calcification due to trauma and psoriasis.

Therapy consists of excision of the excess bone under full aseptic conditions. The nail plate is partially removed and a longitudinal incision is made in the nail bed. The osseous growth with its cartilaginous cap is carefully dissected using fine skin hooks to avoid damage to the fragile nail bed. The tumour is removed with a fine chisel but, whenever possible, the tumour should be removed by an L-shaped or fish-mouth incision, in order to avoid avulsion of the nail plate.

Myxoid pseudocysts of the digits
(Figures 4.25–4.27)

The many synonyms for this lesion reflect its controversial nature: dorsal finger cyst, synovial cyst; recurring myxomatous cyst; cutaneous myxoid cyst; dorsal distal interphalangeal joint ganglion; digital mucinous pseudocyst; focal myxomatous degeneration; mucoid cyst. Whereas some authors regard it as a synovial cyst, most now believe it to be a periarticular degenerative lesion.

Myxoid cysts occur more often in women. They are typically found in the proximal nail fold of the fingers and rarely on toes. The lesions are usually asymptomatic, varying from soft to firm, cystic to fluctuant, and may be dimpled, dome-shaped or smooth-surface. Transillumination confirms their cystic nature. They are always located to one side of the midline and rarely exceed 10 to 15 mm in diameter. The skin over the lesion is thinned and may be verrucous or may even ulcerate. Rarely paronychial fistula may develop beneath the proximal nail fold and exceptionally under the nail plate. Longitudinal grooving of the nail results

from pressure on the matrix. Degenerative, 'wear and tear' osteoarthritis, frequently with Heberden's nodes, is present in most cases.

Histopathology reveals the pseudocystic character. Cavities without synovial lining are located in an ill defined fibrous capsule. The structure is essentially myxomatous with interspersed fibroblasts. Areas of myxomatous degeneration may merge to form a multilocular pseudocyst. In the cavities, a jelly-like substance is found which stains positively for hyaluronic acid. In some cases a mesothelial-like lining is found in the stalk connecting the pseudocyst with the distal interphalangeal joint. It has been suggested that the lesion arises from the joint capsule or tendon sheath synovia, as do ganglia in other areas.

A multitude of treatments have been recommended, including repeated incision and drainage, simple excision, multiple needlings and expression of contents, X-rays (5 Gy, 50 kV, A11 mm, 3 times at weekly intervals), electrocautery, chemical cautery with nitric acid, trichloroacetic acid or phenol, massages or injection of proteolytic substances, hyaluronidase, steroids (flurandrenolone tape, or injections) and sclerosing solutions, freezing with carbon dioxide, radical excision and even amputation.

The intralesional injection of corticosteroid crystal suspension has been recommended. The cyst is first drained from a proximal point to avoid leakage of the steroid suspension when the patient lowers his hand. Careful extirpation of the lesion gives the highest cure rates. A tiny drop of methylene blue solution, diluted with a local anaesthetic and mixed with fresh hydrogen peroxide, is injected into the distal interphalangeal joint at the volar joint crease. The joint will accept only 0.1 to 0.2 ml of dye. This clearly identified the pedicle connecting the joint to the cyst if one is present and also the cyst itself. This procedure sometimes reveals occult satellite cysts. Alternatively the methylene blue may be injected into the cyst to define the tract back to its site of origin. The incision line is drawn on the finger, including a portion of the skin directly over the cyst and continuing proximally in a gentle curve to end dorsally over the joint. The lesion is meticulously dissected from the surrounding soft

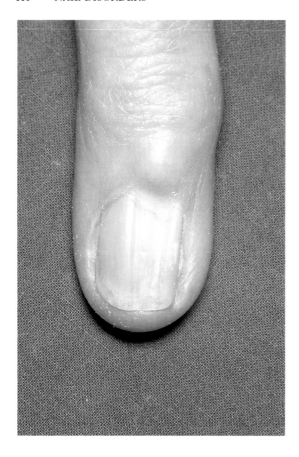

Figure 4.26   Myxoid cyst of index finger with gutter nail deformity.

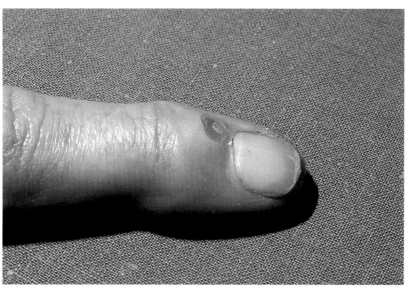

Figure 4.27   Myxoid cyst—erosive type which may get infected; associated here with bony Heberden's nodes.

tissue and the pedicle traced to its origins adjacent to the joint capsule and resected. Dumbbell extension of cysts to each side of the extensor tendon is easily dissected by hyperextending the joint. Osteophytic spurs adjacent to the joint must be removed with a fine chisel or bone rongeur. Recently, liquid nitrogen cryosurgery has been used with an 86 per cent cure rate. The field treated included the cyst and the adjacent proximal area to the transverse skin creases overlying the terminal joint. Two freeze/thaw cycles were carried out, each freeze time being 30 seconds after the ice field had formed, the intervening thaw time being at least 4 minutes; if this method is adopted then longer freeze times must be avoided or permanent matrix damage may occur. For proximal nail fold lesions, excision of the proximal nail folds and associated cyst has been recommended.

Sclerosing agents may also be useful: after puncture and expression of cyst content 0.20–0.30 ml of a 1 per cent solution of sodium tetradecyl sulphate is injected, although a second or a third may be performed at monthly intervals.

Bowen's disease (Figure 4.28)

Bowen's disease represents an intra-epithelial carcinoma. It is not as rare as might appear from the medical literature.

The clinical picture of Bowen's disease of the nail unit is variable. It may form a periungual erythematous, squamous or eroded plaque. In the lateral nail wall and groove, it usually presents as a recalcitrant hyperkeratotic or papillomatous, slowly enlarging lesion. Involvement of the proximal nail fold results in the formation of a characteristic whitish band.

The fingers are far more frequently affected than the toes, typically the thumbs, less often the index and middle fingers. The median age of the patients is about 60 years, males predominating. the development of Bowen's disease is slow. Biopsies taken from the most indurated and warty area often reveal invasive squamous cell carcinoma in contrast to the flat plaque, and therefore

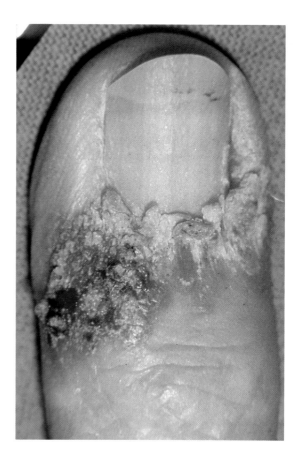

Figure 4.28 Bowen's disease (carcinoma in situ).

many authorities no longer differentiate Bowen's disease from squamous cell carcinoma but use the term epidermoid carcinoma in all cases.

Surgical removal of the affected area and a small margin of 'healthy' tissue is the treatment of choice, some authorities preferring the MOHS fresh tissue removal method.

Squamous cell carcinoma (Figure 4.29)

Squamous cell carcinoma of the nail unit is of low-grade malignancy. Many cases have been

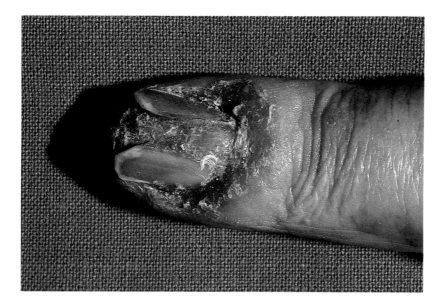

Figure 4.29 Epidermoid (squamous) carcinoma—histology showed some cases still showing carcinoma in-situ.

reported in the literature, with a male predominance. Trauma, chronic infection, and chronic radiation exposure are possible aetiological factors. Two reported cases had associated congenital ectodermal dysplasia. Most occur in the fingers, particularly the thumbs and index fingers.

The presenting symptoms are pain, swelling, inflammation, elevation of the nail, ulceration, tumour mass, ingrowing of the nail, 'pyogenic granuloma' and bleeding. Bone involvement is rare and very late. The duration of symptoms before diagnosis is more than 12 months in over half the cases. Only one case (with ectodermal dysplasia) died from rapid generalized metastases.

Subungual squamous cell carcinoma is slow growing and may be mistaken for chronic infection. This frequent misdiagnosis unduly prolongs the period between the onset of the disease, diagnosis and therapy. Frequently it is not possible to determine whether the cancer was

present initially or developed later, secondary to trauma or infection. As mentioned above, invasive squamous cell carcinoma may develop from Bowen's disease. The possibility of a link with HPV 16, 34 and 35 sheds new light on the aetiology of this type of cancer.

Subungual melanotic lesions (Figures 4.30–4.31)

Melanotic lesions in the subungual region often produce longitudinal nail pigmentation. These light brown to black streaks may be produced by benign melanocytic hyperplasia, lentigo simplex, naevocytic naevus, atypical melanocytic hyperplasia or acral lentiginous melanoma. However, there are many conditions causing brownish to black

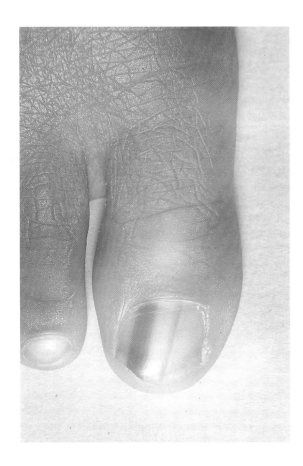

Figure 4.30 Longitudinal melanonychia in a negroid individual. The widened band signifies early malignant melanoma in this case.

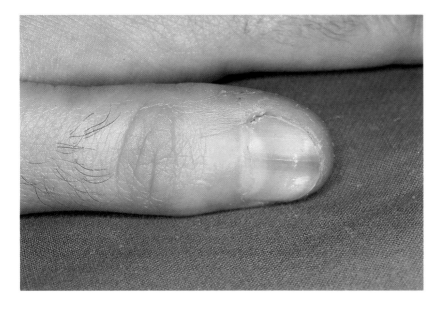

Figure 4.31 Longitudinal melanonychia in Laugier–Hunziker syndrome.

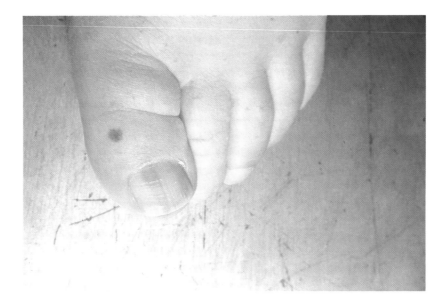

Figure 4.32   Longitudinal melanonychia—acquired; early malignant melanoma.

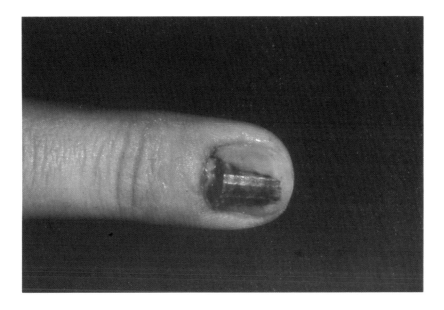

Figure 4.33   Malignant melanoma—broad black band expanded from a line as in Figure 4.32.

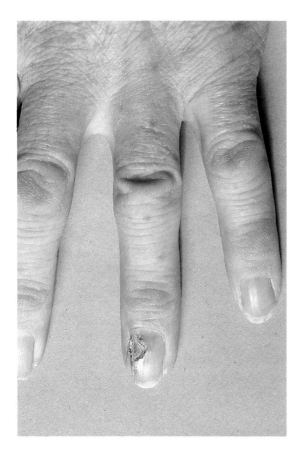

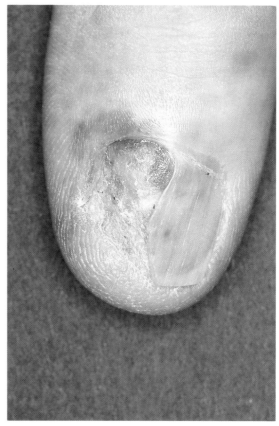

Figure 4.34 Malignant melanoma presenting as a nail dystrophy.

Figure 4.35 Amelanotic malignant melanoma.

discoloration of the nail (see box on page 155), and 25 per cent of subungual melanomata are amelanotic.

Benign melanocytic hyperplasia

This is due to an increased number of relatively normal-looking melanocytes causing a circumscribed hyperpigmented macule in the matrix. Matrix cells become heavily pigmented and retain

their melanin granules throughout the process of nail plate formation, and eventually give rise to a pigmented band. This should be considered a normal phenomenon in pigmented races such as Negroes and Orientals. Longitudinal melanotic streaks are observed in approximately 2.5 per cent of Negro infants, and the incidence progressively increases with age, reaching 96 per cent in blacks over 50 years (Figure 4.30). Melanonychia striata is also common in Japanese with an incidence of from 11 per cent to 23 per cent. In sharp contrast,

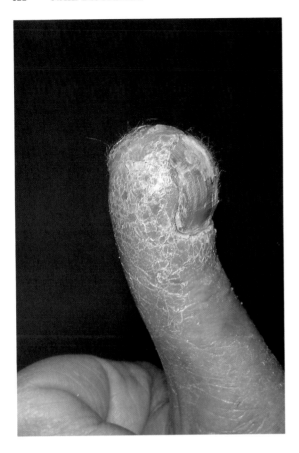

Figure 4.36   Neglected, advanced malignant melanoma.

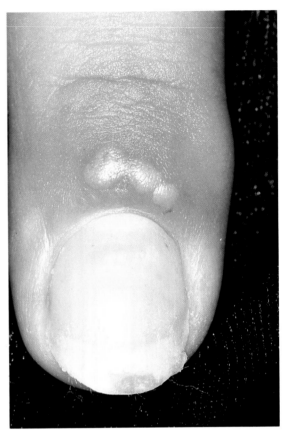

Figure 4.37   Primary herpes simplex—herpetic 'whitlow'.

such melanotic streaks are very rare in Caucasians.

Lentigo simplex and naevocytic naevus

Lentigo simplex is characterized by a considerable increase in highly active melanocytes accompanied by epidermal hyperplasia. The nature of the underlying melanotic lesion responsible for the

pigmented band cannot be determined by clinical examination alone. The same holds true for subungual naevocytic naevi. On histological examination they show nests of naevus cells in the rete ridges with melanin pigmentation of varying intensity. Congenital subungual naevi need excising to exclude secondary malignant melanoma.

Longitudinal brown streaks are also observed in the Laugier–Hunziker syndrome (Figure 4.31). This is characterized by light to dark brown lenticular spots of the buccal and genital mucosa

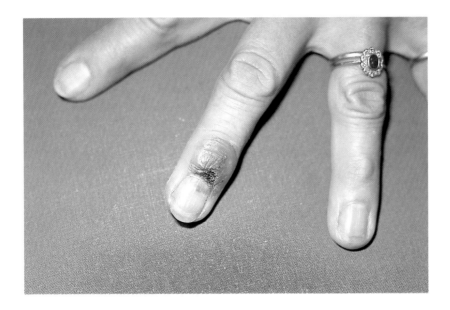

Figure 4.38   Pustulation (bacterial)—late stage; infected myxoid cyst.

associated with melanonychia striata in about one-third of cases. The mucosal pigmented spots are due to an increased number of melanosomes of variable size. No malignant degeneration has been reported.

Atypical melanocytic hyperplasia

Atypical melanocytic hyperplasia shows an increased number of melanocytes with larger, hyperchromatic, pleomorphic nuclei, more prominent nucleoli, increased mitoses, and long branching dendrites. Thus, atypical melanocytic hyperplasia may be considered to be incipient malignant melanoma.

The outcome of benign subungual pigmented lesions is not fully known. Benign melanocytic hyperplasia may develop into lentigo simplex, which may be a forerunner of a naevocytic naevus.

Malignant melanomas in other anatomical sites are known to arise both in naevocytic naevi and atypical melanocytic hyperplasia, and the first subungual malignant melanoma ever described as 'fongus hématodes' developed from a pigmented lesion that had been present for 28 years. Similar reports have appeared in the literature, strongly suggesting that every pigmented subungual lesion in a Caucasian must be biopsied, preferably by a complete excision either as active melanoma prophylaxis or as therapy for an already malignant melanoma.

Malignant melanoma (Figures 4.32–4.36)

In the nail apparatus the most common initial sign is acquired longitudinal melanonychia in white Caucasians or broadening of an existing band in oriental or negroid individuals. This tumour and its practical differential diagnosis from other chromonychias and nail dystrophies is described here, though linear melanonychia from other causes is considered in Chapter 6.

Melanoma of the nail region is now better understood since the identification and analysis of acrolentiginous melanoma. It may be localized subungually or periungually with pigmentation and/or dystrophy of the nail plate. Initial lesions may be mistaken histologically for benign or atypical melanocytic hyperplasia, but serial sections usually reveal the true nature of the disease.

Approximately 2 to 3 per cent of melanomas in Caucasians, and 15 to 20 per cent in blacks, are located in the nail unit. However, malignant melanoma is rare in Negroes, and therefore the number of ungual melanomas in Caucasians and Negroes does not significantly differ. In Caucasians, most patients have a fair complexion, light hair, and blue or hazel eyes. There is no sex predominance, though some reports favour female, others male predominance. The mean age is 55 to 60 years. Most tumours are found in the thumbs or great toes.

Melanoma of the nail region is often asymptomatic. Many patients only notice a pigmented lesion after trauma to the area; only approximately two-thirds seek medical advice because of the appearance of the lesion. Pain or discomfort is rare, and nail deformity, spontaneous ulceration, sudden change in colour, bleeding or tumour mass breaking through the nail are even more infrequent.

It is useful to remember that a pigmented subungual lesion is more likely to be malignant than benign. If the melanoma is pigmented it may show one or more of the following characteristics:
a) A spot, which appears in the matrix, nail bed or plate. This may vary in colour from brown to black: it may be homogenous or irregular and is seldom painful.
b) A longitudinal brown to black band of variable width running through the whole visible nail.
c) Less frequently, but almost pathognomonic, a brown to black discoloration spreads from under the nail or proximal nail bed to the surrounding skin. This phenomenon is termed 'Hutchinson's

sign' and has proved to be a valuable clue to the clinical diagnosis of malignance. Its presence means that the entire nail apparatus must be removed (without prior incisional biopsy). This technique enables serial sections to be examined, which is particularly important in acral lentiginous melanoma in which histology may be difficult to interpret. Very rarely, periungual hyperpigmentation may be seen in melanocytic lesions other than malignant melanoma, such as in naevocytic naevus and Laugier–Hunziker syndrome (usually involving several nails).

The nail plate may also become thickened or fissured and permanently shed.

Approximately 25 per cent of the melanomas are amelanotic and may mimic pyogenic granuloma, granulation tissue, or ingrowing nail. The risk of misdiagnosis is particularly high in these cases.

Malignant melanoma must be considered in the differential diagnosis (see box on page 126) in all cases of inexplicable chronic paronychia, whether painful or not, in torpid granulomatous ulceration of the proximal nail fold, and in pseudoverrucous keratotic alterations of the nail bed and lateral nail groove. Subungual melanoma may also simulate mycobacterial infections, mycotic onychodystrophy, recalcitrant paronychia, and ingrowing nail. Subungual haematoma is not rare and may present without a history of severe trauma. It may follow repeated minor trauma which escapes the patient's attention, such as in 'tennis toe', or follow trauma from hard ski boots. Although haematoma following a single trauma usually grows out in one piece rather than as a longitudinal streak, due to the continuous production of pigment, repeated trauma may cause difficulties in differential diagnosis. It is recommended that the lesion should be examined with a magnifying loup after it has been covered by a drop of oil. The pigmented nail should be clipped and tested with the argentaffin reaction in order to rule out melanin pigmentation. Subungual haemoglobin is not degraded to haemosiderin and is therefore Prussian blue-negative. Scrapings or small pieces of the nail boiled with water in a test tube give a positive benzidine reaction with the conventional haemostix.

The difference between haemosiderinic and melanotic pigment, sometimes rather difficult to discern by routine histological methods, is easily seen by ultrastructural techniques: ferrous pigment is intercellular while melanin is intracellular.

Because of its frequency, melanonychia striata in deeply pigmented races is considered a normal finding, but up to one-fifth of all melanomas in blacks are in the subungual area, and these typically begin with a pigmented spot producing a longitudinal streak. These spots are usually black rather than the normal brown. The diagnosis may be aided by comparing them with the brown stripes in other nails or by the occurrence of Hutchinson's sign.

Histological examination of acral lentiginous melanoma requires great experience, and often serial sections are needed to classify the lesion accurately. Grading according to Clark's levels or Breslow's maximum tumour thickness is difficult and often inconclusive.

Subungual melanoma has a poor prognosis. The reported 5-year survival rates are from 35 to 50 per cent. Most patients present with advanced subungual melanoma; however, even early diagnosis is not a guarantee of a good prognosis. Women have a better prognosis than men.

Factors which contribute to a poor prognosis are delay in diagnosis and, as a result of this, inadequate treatment. The tumour may be mistaken for a sequel to trauma, and valuable time may be lost before the diagnosis is made. Treatment depends on the stage of the disease. Level I and Level II melanomas may be adequately treated by wide local excision, and repair of the defect with graft or flap. Amputation is usually advised for melanoma at levels more advanced than II. When the thumb is affected and therefore amputated, pollicization of a finger may provide a functional replacement. There would appear to be no relationship between the prognosis and the extent of the amputation, though metacarpo/metatarsophalangeal amputation is considered to be inadequate because of local recurrences. The rationale for elective lymph node dissection and/or isolated hyperthermic

Range of tumours and swellings affecting the nail apparatus (those underlined described in the text)

Warts
Verrucous epidermal naevus
Subungual papilloma
Verrucous lesions in incontinentia pigmenti
Subungual corn
Epidermoid cyst
Fibromata
   Keloids
   'True' fibroma
   Koenen's tumour
   Acquired periungual fibrokeratoma
   Subungual filamentous tumour
   Benign juvenile digital fibromatosis
Leiomyoma
Benign synovialoma
Xanthoma
Lipoma
Neurogenic tumours
Multicentric reticulohistocytosis (see Chapter 7)
Actinic keratosis
Arsenical keratosis
Glomus tumour
Pyogenic granuloma
Naevus flammeus and angioma
Angiokeratoma circumscriptum
Aneurysmal bone cyst (arteriovenous fistula)
Subungual exostosis
Enchondroma
   Maffucci's syndrome
Osteoid osteoma
Hereditary multiple exostosis (diaphysial aclasis)
Myxoid pseudocyst
Myxoma
Bowen's disease
Squamous cell carcinoma
Keratoacanthoma
Basal cell carcinoma
Sarcoma
Kaposi's sarcoma
Lymphoma
Metastases
Melanotic/Melanocytic lesions
   Benign melanocytic hyperplasia
   Lentigo simplex and naevocytic naevus
   Atypoical melanocytic hyperplasia
   Peutz–Jeghers–Touraine syndrome
   Malignant melanoma
   Laugier–Hunziker syndrome

perfusion of the extremity with cytotoxic drugs is still under discussion. Immune enhancement such as BCG therapy is used in some centres.

Tumours of the nail unit (by site)

At the nail fold/plate junction	Acquired periungual fibrokeratoma
	Periungual fibroma (tuberose sclerosis)
Within the nail fold	Myxoid pseudocysts
	Tendon sheath giant cell tumour (ganglion)
	Verruca vulgaris
	Metastases
Within the nail bed with or without nail plate destruction	Subungual exostosis
	Osteochondroma
	Enchondroma
	Subungual corn
	Pyogenic granuloma
	Glomus tumour
	Recurring digital fibrous tumour of childhood
	Bowen's disease and squamous cell carcinoma
	Melanoma
	Metastases

Differential diagnosis of subungual malignant melanoma

Malignant lesions | *Benign lesions*

Pigmented

Haemangioendothelioma
Kaposi's sarcoma
Metastatic melanoma

Melanonychia striata (Chapter 6) due to:
Melanocytic hyperplasia
Junctional naevi
Adrenal insufficiency
Adrenalectomy for Cushing's Disease
Angiokeratoma
Chromogenic bacteria (Proteus)
Drugs: antimalarials, cytotoxics, arsenic, silver, thallium, phenothiazines and PUVA
Haematoma, trauma
Irradiation
Laugier–Hunziker syndrome
Onychomycosis nigricans

Amelanotic

Basal cell carcinoma
Bowen's disease
Metastasis
Squamous cell carcinoma

Epidermal cyst
Exostosis
Foreign body granuloma
Keratoacanthoma
Pyogenic granuloma
Unguis incarnatus

Pustules (Figures 4.37–4.45)

The conditions in which nail apparatus pustulation may be a significant sign are listed in the box on page 135.

Herpes simplex (Figure 4.37)

Distal digital herpes simplex infection may affect the terminal phalanx as a herpetic 'whitlow' or start as an acute, intensely painful, paronychia. It is relatively common in dental staff, anaesthetists and those involved with the care of the mouth and upper respiratory tract in unconscious patients. Recurrent forms are generally less severe and have a milder clinical course than the initial infection.

After an incubation period of 3–7 days during which local tenderness, erythema and swelling may develop, a crop of vesicles appears at the portal of entry into the skin. The vesicles typically are distributed in the paronychia and on the volar digital skin, resembling pyogenic infection of the fingertip.

Close inspection, however, will reveal the classic pale, raised vesicles surrounded by an erythematous border. An acutely painful whitlow may develop and extend under the distal free edge of the nail and into the nail bed. A distinct predilection for the thumb, index and ring fingers on the dominant hand has been noted, but any finger may be involved. Multiple lesions are rare. For 10–14 days the vesicles gradually increase in size, often coalescing into large, honeycombed bullae. New crops of lesions may appear during this time. Vesicular fluid is clear early in the disease but may become turbid, seropurulent or even haemorrhagic within days of onset. At times, a pale yellow colour of the vesicles will suggest pyogenic infection, yet frank pus is not usually obtained. Patients complain of tenderness and severe throbbing in the affected digit. Coexisting primary herpetic infections of the mouth and fingernails suggest autoinoculation of the virus into the nail tissues as a result of nail-biting or finger-sucking.

Radiating pain along the C7 distribution is sometimes noted preceding each recurrent attack. Lymphangitis may start from the wrist and extend to the axilla with enlarged and tender lymph nodes. Numbness and hypoaesthesia following the acute episode has been observed.

The diagnosis of herpetic infection can be made readily by examining the base of the vesicles for the characteristic multinucleated 'balloon' giant cells, in stained smears. The presence of intranuclear inclusions is also significant. Viral cultivation is confirmatory and is usually positive within 24 hours on onset; the active viral phase is up to 4–5 days in primary attacks but only 2–3 days in recurrent episodes.

Differential diagnosis

It is important to exclude primary or recurrent herpes simplex infection in the differential diagnosis of every vesiculopustular finger infection. The typical appearance of the lesions with disproportionate intensity of the pain, the absence of pus in the confluent multiloculated vesiculopustular lesions and the lack of increased tension in the finger pulp aid in distinguishing this slow healing infection from a bacterial foreign body or paronychia (contrast 4.38).

Herpes zoster infections, which may affect the proximal nail fold like herpes simplex, also involve the entire sensory dermatome. The pustules of primary cutaneous *Neisseria gonorrhoeae* infection may resemble herpes simplex on the rare occasion when it occurs on the finger. The diagnosis is established by Gram stain and bacteriological confirmation.

Treatment is aimed primarily at symptomatic relief and the avoidance of secondary infection. Topical acyclover may shorten the course of any one attack; given orally the drug may prevent recurrences whilst it is being taken. On cessation of the treatment relapses are unfortunately common. This is a preventable infection. Gloves should always be worn on both hands for procedures such as intubation, removal of dentures or providing oral care, despite the additional costs involved.

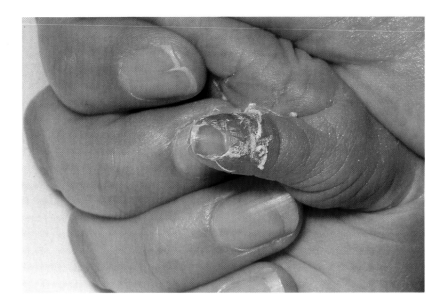

Figure 4.39   Infantile impetigo.

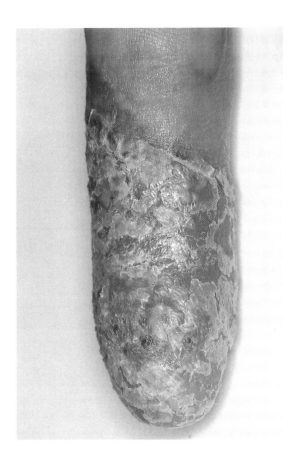

Figure 4.40   Acropustulosis; of psoriatic type.

Subungual infection in the newborn due to Veillonella

Many epidemics of subungual infection have been described among infants in postnatal wards and special care baby units. The number of fingers affected per patient ranged from one to ten; the thumbs are less frequently involved than other fingers, and the toe nails are spared altogether. Three stages occur: firstly, a small amount of clear fluid appears under the centre of the nail, along with mild inflammation at the distal end of the finger. This initial vesicle lasts approximately 24 hours; it sometimes enlarges but never to the edge of the nail. Some small lesions bypass the second, pustular stage, going directly to the third stage. As a rule the fluid becomes yellow after 24 hours, the pus remaining for 24–48 hours before gradually turning brown, and being absorbed. This colour fades progressively over a period of 2 to 6 weeks, leaving the nail and nail bed apparently completely normal.

Subungual pus obtained by aseptic puncture of the nails showed tiny, Gram-negative cocci about $0.4\,\mu m$ in diameter. These organisms resemble *Veillonella*, a group of anaerobes of dubious pathogenicity found as commensals in the saliva, vagina, and respiratory tract. Systemic antibiotics did not change the clinical course of the nail lesions which did not differ from those observed in other untreated and affected newborn children.

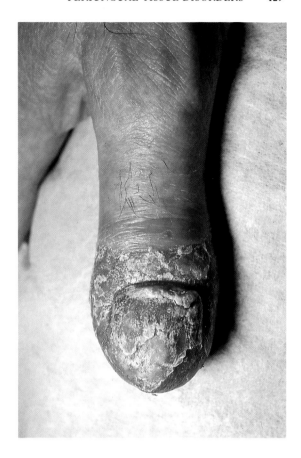

Figure 4.41   Pustular psoriasis—this patient previously had chronic psoriasis vulgaris.

Impetigo (Figure 4.39)

The dorsal aspect of the distal phalanx may be involved by impetigo. It comes in two forms: 1) vesiculopustular, with its familiar honey-crusted lesions, usually due to β-haemolytic streptococci; 2) bullous, usually due to phage type 71 staphylococci. The latter is characterized by the appearance of large, localized, intraepidermal bullae that persist for longer periods than the transient vesicles of streptococcal impetigo which subsequently rupture spontaneously to form very thin crusts.

The lesions of bullous impetigo may mimic the non-infectious bullous diseases (such as drug-induced or pemphigoid). Oral therapy of bullous impetigo with a penicillinase-resistant penicillin should be instituted and continued until the lesions resolve. Cephalexin and erythromycin are acceptable substitutes. The lesions should be cleansed several times daily and topical aureomycin (3 per cent) applied to all the affected areas.

Blistering distal dactylitis

Blistering distal dactylitis (BDD) is a variant of streptococcal skin infection. It presents as a superficial, tender, blistering β-haemolytic streptococcal infection over the anterior fat pad of the distal phalanx of the finger. The lesion may or may not have a paronychial extension. This blister, containing thin, white pus, has a predilection for the tip of the digit and extends to the subungual area of the free edge of the nail plate. The area may provide a nidus for the β-haemolytic streptococcus and act as a focus of chronic infection similar to the nasopharynx. The age range of affected patients is 2 to 16 years. For local care incision, drainage and antiseptic soaking are indicated and facilitate a more rapid response to systemic antibiotic therapy: effective regimes include benzathine penicillin G in a single intramuscular dose, or a 10-day course of oral phenoxymethylpenicillin or erythromycin ethyl succinate. This type of treatment decreases the reservoir of streptococci by preventing spread to family contacts. It has been described as an infective complication of ingrowing toe nail.

The differential diagnosis includes blisters resulting from friction, thermal and chemical burns, infectious states such as herpetic whitlow and staphylococcal bullous impetigo and the Weber–Cokayne variant of epidermolysis bullosa simplex.

Gonorrhoea

The hallmark of disseminated gonococcaemia is its skin lesions. The most common is the vesicopustule which occurs juxta-articularly over the extensor surfaces of the hands, and dorsal surfaces of the toes and around the nails. Haemorrhagic bullae occur in small numbers but in the same area. A further skin manifestation is focal petechiae over the digits or the medial aspects of the ankles.

Primary extragenital cutaneous gonorrhoea acquired in a venereal fashion is extremely rare. It presents with a fingertip abcess extending under the nail plate with peripheral erythema to the pustular lesion. The diagnosis of gonococcal skin infection is often not entertained until the unexpected findings on the Gram stain examination prompts further questioning and bacteriological confirmation.

Self-inflicted bullous lesions

This bullous eruption in the newborn infant is always present from the time of birth, beginning in utero. It may appear on the dorsum of the thumb or along the dorsal aspect of the index finger. The bullae measure from 0.5 cm to 1.5 cm in diameter and contain fluid of clear consistency and light yellow colour. Bacterial cultures show no growth. These lesions are presumed to be self-inflicted (in utero) as a consequence of a vigorous sucking reflex in otherwise normal newborns. The differential diagnosis includes epidermolysis bullosa, incontinentia pigmenti and congenital syphilis. Staphylococcal and streptococcal bullae generally do not occur before the fifth day of life, and vesicular eruptions due to herpes simplex do not occur before the sixth day.

Chronic paronychia and thumb-sucking

Candida paronychia, usually in association with oral candidosis, may arise as a result of chronic maceration due to thumb-sucking.

Chronic paronychia is not uncommon in children. It differs from the condition seen in adults in the source of the maceration, associated diseases, the clinical appearances of the lesion, and the patients' responses to the symptoms. In children the lesions are generally very prominent, with total involvement of the proximal nail fold. The skin is usually erythematous and glistening due to the wet environment produced by continuous thumb sucking. The quality of the nail substance is regularly altered, making its texture poor. The habit of sucking fingers or thumbs is the most important predisposing factor. Candida *albicans* is present in all cases. When an acute flare-up occurs the patient experiences pruritus and discomfort in the proximal nail fold. Children respond to this by sucking, the symptoms of chronic paronychia perpetuating the habit which intiated the maceration. The lesions tend to be more severe in childhood than in adult paronychia probably because thumb-sucking is more continuous than exposure to wet work, and saliva is more irritating than water. The minor repeated trauma resulting from suction is capable of causing complete loss of the nail plate. Detection of the carrier state in the mouth and gastrointestinal tract by cultures of saliva and stools may be important in the occasional patient with refractory paronychia. Persistent and repeated candida paronychia in infancy suggests a more serious underlying disorder and such infants should be investigated for endocrine disease and immune deficiency syndromes.

Thumb- or finger-sucking is sometimes associated with herpes simplex. This may result in localized extensions of the eruption producing a viral stomatitis combined with involvement of the digit.

In childhood, local trauma, caused by onychophagia, may result in the development of opportunistic infection by the normal oropharyngeal flora, amongst which are found HB 1 bacteria. Acute paronychia may also be caused by HB 1 organisms (*Eikenella corrodens*), but it is uncommon in the absence of an immune deficiency.

Acropustuloses/pustular psoriasis (Figures 4.40–4.42)

In pustular psoriasis and acrodermatitis continua, involvement of a single digit is common. It is often misdiagnosed when the pustule appears beneath the nail plate with necrosis of tissue resulting in dessication and crust formation. New pustule formation may develop at the periphery or within the lesions. The nail is lifted off by the crust and lakes of pus and new pustules may form on the denuded nail bed. Permanent loss is possible.

Acral pustular psoriasis has been reported with resorptive osteolysis ('deep Koebner phenomenon') and pronounced skin and subcutaneous tissue atrophy. There may be progressive loss of entire digits in the feet and loss of fingertips and fingernails. 'Tuft' osteolysis may occur independently of acropustuloses and arthritis. Histopathology reveals Munro–Sabouraud 'microabscesses' or the spongiform pustule of Kogoj.

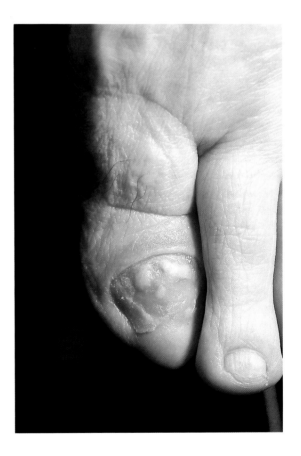

Figure 4.42 Nail bed pustulation after nail shedding—pustular psoriasis.

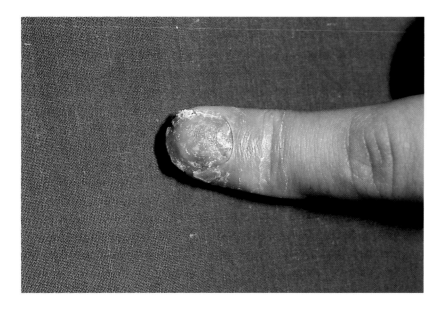

Figure 4.43   Severe dystrophic parakeratosis pustulosa.

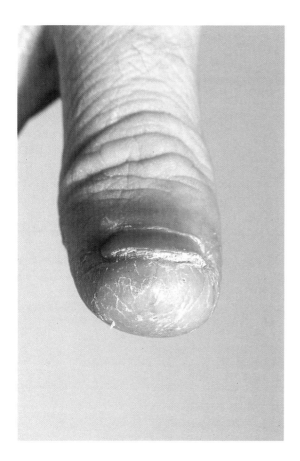

Figure 4.44   Parakeratosis pustulosa; less acute than in Figure 4.43 and very little nail dystrophy.

Localized PUVA can be of benefit. Oral retinoid therapy may give good short-term results; but recurrences appear 1 to 3 months after the treatment has been stopped. Combined retinoid and PUVA treatment delays and lowers the frequency of relapse. Topical mechloretamine has given some good results as has intramuscular triamcinolone acetonide.

The differential diagnosis of acropustulosis may be controversial, particularly with regard to the subcorneal pustula dermatosis of Sneddon and Wilkinson. Many authorities have described patients with pustular lesions like those described as subcorneal pustular dermatosis, but who had in addition stigmata suggestive of psoriasis. These included typical scaly plaques on the elbows and knees, pitted nails or arthropathy. It is, however, pointless to debate the pathogenesis of Sneddon–Wilkinson disease without applying the techniques available for identifying the psoriatic state: cell kinetics, complement activation in the stratum corneum, HLA/family studies, and nail growth studies.

Reiter's syndrome

The clinical and histological features of the skin changes in patients with Reiter's syndrome may be indistinguishable from those of patients with psoriasis. Skin changes resembling paronychia can accompany nail involvement suggesting inflammation of the proximal nail fold. Onycholysis, ridging, splitting, greenish-yellow or sometimes brownish-red discoloration and subungual hyperkeratosis may be present. Small yellow pustules may develop and slowly enlarge beneath the nail, often near the lunula. Their contents become dry and brown. The nails may be shed. Nail pitting may be seen in Reiter's syndrome, individual pits being deep and punched out. This nail pitting may reflect a predisposition to the development of psoriasis or psoriasiform lesions dependent on the HLA-A^2 and B 27 antigens, as suggested by previously reported HLA typing studies. HLA-A^2 and B 27 were present in a 6-year-old boy who had only the nail changes which were compatible with Reiter's syndrome; the same antigens were also present in his father, who had uveitis, arthritis, and amyloidosis.

Antibiotics, steroids and nonsteroidal anti-inflammatory drugs are without benefit. PUVA may be helpful. Oral retinoid therapy may clear the nails in Reiter's syndrome. Combined chemotherapy with methotrexate, oral retinoid and prednisolone has been suggested.

Parakeratosis pustulosa (Figures 4.43–4.45)

This parakeratotic condition of the fingertip was first described more than 50 years ago. It usually occurs in girls of approximately 7 years of age, typically affecting only one digit, usually a finger. The lesions start close to the free margin of the nail of a finger or toe. In some cases, a few isolated pustules or vesicles may be observed in the initial phase; these usually disappear before the patient presents to the doctor. Confluent eczematoid changes cover the skin immediately adjacent to the distal edge of the nail. The affected area is pink or of normal skin colour and densely studded with fine scales; there is a clear margin between the normal and affected areas. The skin changes may extend to the dorsal aspect of the finger or toe, but usually only the fingertip is affected. The most striking and characteristic change is the hyperkeratosis beneath the nail tip. The nail plate is lifted up, deformed and often thickened. Commonly the deformity produced is asymmetrical and limited to one corner of the distal edge, or at least more pronounced at the corners of the nail. Pitting occurs in some cases; rarely transverse ridging of the nail plate is present. Most cases resolve within a few months, but some cases persist for many years, even into adult life.

Histological findings are of some value, including hyperkeratosis and parakeratosis, pustulation and crusts; acanthosis and mild exocytosis, papillomatosis and heavy cellular infiltrates composed mainly of lymphocytes and fibroblasts around dilated capillary loops. This histology

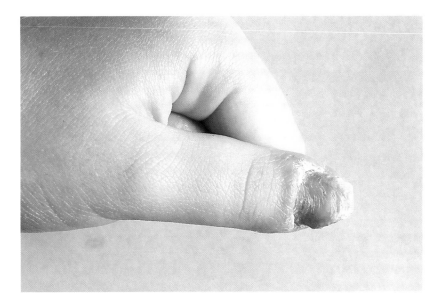

Figure 4.45   Parakeratosis pustulosa with nail hypertrophy and nail bed hyperkeratosis.

presents many of the features common to psoriasis and eczema.

In the differential diagnosis of parakeratosis pustulosa, the following points are important:

- Pustules are very rare and only seen in the initial stage, as distinct from pustular psoriasis or acropustulosis.

- Patients with psoriasis develop a coarse sheet of scales and not the fine type of scaling typically seen in parakeratosis pustolosa.

- The age distribution differs from that found in atopic dermatitis which may cause transverse ridging due to the involvement of the proximal nail fold.

- If the nail changes predominate, especially on a toe, the disorder can be mistaken for onychomycosis. Thumb-sucking, which is a predisposing factor in chronic candidal paronychia, should be ruled out when a single thumb is affected.

No treatment makes any difference to the frequency of recurrence or the overall duration of parakeratosis pustulosa. Topical steroids provide some symptomatic relief.

Acrokeratosis paraneoplastica of Bazex and Dupré

Acrokeratosis paraneoplastica occurs in association with malignant epithelial tumours of the upper respiratory or digestive tracts, in particular the pharyngolaryngeal area—pyriform fossa, tonsillar area, epiglottis, hard and soft palate, vocal cords, tongue, lower lip, oesophagus and the upper third of the lungs. It also occurs with metastases to the cervical and upper mediastinal lymph nodes. This 'paraneoplasia' may precede the signs of the associated malignancy, disappear when the tumour is removed and reappear with its recurrence; however, the nail involvement does not always benefit from total recovery, in contrast to the other lesions. This condition almost exclusively occurs in men over 40 years of age. The lesions are erythematous and keratotic with ill-defined borders. They are symmetrically distributed, affecting hands, feet, ears and occasionally the nose. The two nails suffer more severely than the finger nails. Roughened, irregular, keratotic, fissured and warty excrescences are found equally on the terminal phalanges of both fingers and toes.

The nails are invariably involved and are typically the earliest manifestation of the disease. In mild forms, the nail involvement is discrete; the affected nails are thin, soft and may become fragile and crumble. In more established disease, the nails are flaky, irregular, whitened and the free edge is raised by subungual hyperkeratosis.

In severe forms, the lesions resemble advanced psoriatic nail dystrophy and may progress to complete loss of the diseased nails. The nail bed is eventually replaced by a smooth epidermis to which the irregular, horny vestiges of the nail still adhere. The periungual skin shows an erythematosquamous eruption, predominantly on the dorsum of the terminal phalanges, and there may be associated chronic paronychia with occasional, acute suppurative exacerbations.

The two extremes of the disease may coexist. In these cases, the proximal third of the nail is atrophic and the distal two-thirds exhibits hypertrophic changes. The histopathological changes are non-specific, though they do enable the exclusion of psoriasis, lupus erythematosus or other similar eruptions.

Further reading

Paronychia

Baran R and **Bureau H,** Congenital malalignment of the big toe-nail as a cause of ingrowing toe-nail in infancy. Pathology and treatment (a study of thirty cases). *Clin Exp Dermatol* (1983) **8**:619–23.

Barth JH and **Dawber RPR,** Diseases of the nails in children. *Pediatr Dermatol* (1987) **4**:275–90.

Editorial, Chronic paronychia. *Brit Med J* (1975) **ii**:460.

Tumours and swellings

Briggs JC, Subungual malignant melanoma: a review article. *Br J Plast Surg* (1985) **38**:174–6.

Salasche SJ and **Garland LD,** Tumors of the nail. *Dermatol Clin* (1985) **3**:501–19.

Pustules

Hjorth N and **Thomsen K,** Parakeratosis pustulosa. *Br J Dermatol* (1967) **79**:527–32.

Conditions in which nail pustulation may occur	
Infective (primary cause)	Acute paronychia (see Chapter 4) Blistering distal dactylitis Hand–foot–mouth disease Herpes simplex (primary and recurrent) Gonorrhoea Impetigo *Veillonella* infection—newborn
Non-infective (secondary infection may occur)	Ingrowing toe nail Malalignment in childhood Common type Self-inflicted bullous lesions of newborn Thumb-sucking (and paronychia)
Dermatoses	Acrokeratosis paraneoplastica Acropustulosis/psoriasis Parakeratosis pustulosa Reiter's syndrome

5

Nail consistency

Fragile, brittle and soft nails (Figures 5.1–5.8)

Many nail diseases which disrupt nail formation and structure will lead to 'secondary' brittleness and fragility. In this chapter only those conditions leading to nail fragility or brittleness as a main complaint are considered in any detail.

'Hapalonychia' is the term used for soft nail in which there is no primary specific local nail disease to explain it. Diseases and conditions associated with this include: congenital types, sulphur deficiency syndromes, thin nail plate of any cause, occupational disease (for example working with industrial oils), chronic arthritis leprosy, hypothyroidism, peripheral ischaemia, peripheral neuritis, hemiplegia and cachexic states.

In some cases of hapalonychia the thinned nails assumed a semi-transparent, bluish-white hue, sometimes described as 'egg-shell nails'.

Brittle nails can be divided into four main types on morphological grounds:

● An isolated split at the free edge which sometimes extends proximally. This may result from onychorrhexis with its shallow parallel furrows running in the superficial layer of the nail.

● Multiple, crenellated splitting which resembles the battlements of a castle. Triangular pieces may easily be torn from the free margin.

● A lamellar splitting of the free edge of the nail into fine layers. It may occur in isolation or associated with the other types.

● Transverse splitting and breaking of the lateral edge close to the distal margin.

The changes in brittle, friable nails are often confined to the surface of the nail plate; this occurs in superficial white onychomycosis and may be seen after the application of nail polish or base coat which causes 'granulations' in the nail keratin. In advanced psoriasis and fungal infection the friability may extend throughout the entire nail.

The changes in nail consistency may be due to impairment of one or more of the factors on which the health of the nail depends, such as variations in the water content or keratin structures. In addition, changes in the intercellular structures, cell membranes, and intracellular changes in the arrangement of keratin fibrils have been revealed by electron microscopy. Normal nails contain approximately 18 per cent water. After prolonged immersion in water this percentage is increased and the nail becomes soft; this makes toe nail trimming and nail biopsies much easier. A low lipid content may decrease the nail's ability to retain water. If the water content is considerably reduced, the nail becomes brittle. Splitting, which results from this brittle quality, is probably partly due to repeated uptake and drying-out of water.

The keratin content may be modified by chemical and physical insults, especially in occupational nail disorders. Amino-acid chains may be broken or distorted by alkalis, oxidizing agents and thioglycolates, such as chemicals employed in the permanent waving processes. These break or distort the multiple S–S bond linkages which join the protein chains to form the keratin fibrils. Keratin structure can also be changed in genetic disorders, such as dyskeratosis congenita in which the nail plate is completely absent, or reduced to thin, dystrophic remnants.

The composition of the nail plate is sometimes related to generalized disease. High sulphur content in the form of cystine predominates, which contributes to the stability of the fibrous protein by the formation of disulphide bonds. A lack of iron can result in softening of the nail and koilonychia; conversely, the calcium content in the nail would appear to contribute little towards its hardness. Calcium is mainly in the surface of the nail, in small absorbed quantities, and X-ray defraction shows no evidence of calcite or apatite crystals. Damage to both the central and peripheral nervous system may result in nail fragility.

Factors leading to fragile, brittle or soft nails (Figures 5.1–5.8)

Local factors	Trauma
	Alopecia areata
	Chemical
	Alkalis/oxidizing agents
	Detergents
	Industrial oils
	Nail cosmetic procedures, eg varnishes
	Solvents
	Thioglycolates
	Water (hydration–dehydration effects)
	Conditions which thin the nail plate
	Darier's disease (Figure 5.3)
	Lichen planus (Figures 5.1, 5.2)
	Psoriasis (Figure 5.4)
	Slow nail growth
General factors	Arsenic poisoning
	Cachexic states
	Chronic arthropathies (fingers or toes)
	Iron deficiency
	Neurological
	Hemiplegia
	Neuropathies
	Oral retinoids (Figure 5.6)
	Osteoporosis/osteomalacia
	Peripheral circulatory impairment (arterial) (Figures 5.7, 5.8)
	Sulphur deficiency diseases
	Systemic amyloidosis
	Vitamin A, C and B6 deficiencies

Causes of nail fragility

These may be local or, less frequently, systemic (see box).

Local causes

The nail may be damaged by trauma or by chemical agents such as detergents, alkalis, various solvents and sugar solutions and especially by hot water.

The nail plate requires 5–6 months in order to regenerate and therefore it is vulnerable to daily insults. The housewife is very susceptible; particularly at risk are the first three fingers of the dominant hand. Anything which slows the rate of nail growth will increase the risk. Cosmetic causes are rare. Some varnishes will damage the superficial layers of the nail. Drying may be enhanced by some nail varnish removers and soaking fingers in a warm soapy solution, for removing the cuticle, is especially dangerous; this is common practice among manicurists. It has been shown that climatic and seasonal factors may affect the hydration of the nail plate.

Fragility, due to thinning of the nail plate, may be caused by a reduction in the length of the matrix. Diminution, or even complete arrest of nail formation over a variable width may be the result of many dermatoses such as eczema, lichen planus, psoriasis (rare) and impairment of the peripheral circulation. The frequency of nail fragility in alopecia areata lends credence to the popular belief that nail and hair disorders are often associated.

General causes

These are listed in the box on page 138. The diverse constituents of the nail plate, especially the enzymes necessary for the formation of keratin, are subject to genetic influences and changes in them are manifested in the form of hereditary disease.

Treatment of brittle nails

Moisture (excess hydration) and trauma must be avoided at all costs; routine household chores are particularly damaging. Protection with rubber gloves worn over light cotton glove liners should be used in order to avoid direct contact with water.

Systemic treatment may be helpful. Oral iron, even in the absence of demonstrable iron deficiency (given for 6 months) may be of some value. The following regime has been suggested but with no objective proof of its efficacy: evening primrose oil, 2 capsules tid, pyridoxine 25–30 mg per day and ascorbic acid 2–3 g per day. Recently, biotin has been shown to improve the quality of horse hoofs, pig claws and — possibly — human nails.

Brittle nails tested with a standardized micrometric method, swell significantly less than normal nails: an increase of this 'swelling factor' was seen in 10 patients treated with a mixture of thiamin, calcium-D-panthothenate, L-cystine and p-aminobenzoic acid; gelatin was found to be inefficient.

Since it takes several months for the finger nails to be completely replaced, some authorities suggest such treatment as small doses of oral vitamin A, which beneficially affect keratinization. Warm environment and hyperaemia may also lead to faster growth, thus giving a reduction in the time the nail plate is exposed to repeated minor chemical and physical action which accentuate nail fragility.

There is no efficient barrier cream able to prevent over-softening of the nails due to water and detergents. After hydration, the nail plate should be massaged with mineral oil or a lubricating cream to prevent the nail from drying out. Under experimental conditions hydration may be further enhanced by the addition of phospholipids which have been shown to be effective in increasing and maintaining the increased nail flexibility. This may result from an occlusive effect of the applications which may delay the evaporation of water. Base coat, nail polish and hard top coat act in a similar manner and also have a splint-like effect in strengthening the nail.

Soft nails may be hardened by painting them daily with 5 per cent aluminium chloride in propylene glycol and water.

Further reading

Fragile, brittle and soft nails

Kechijian P, Brittle fingernails. *Dermatol Clin* (1985) **3**:421–9.

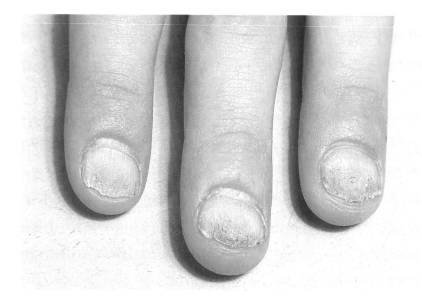

Figure 5.1 Fragile, brittle nails, with softening and koilonychia—lichen planus '20 nail dystrophy'.

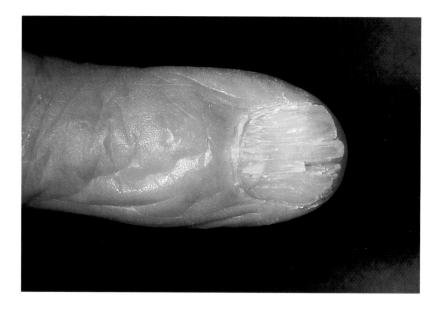

Figure 5.2 Lichen planus fragility of nails.

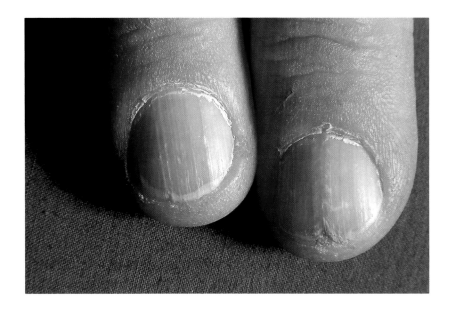

Figure 5.3 Darier's disease—distal focal fragility due to linear keratinization defect.

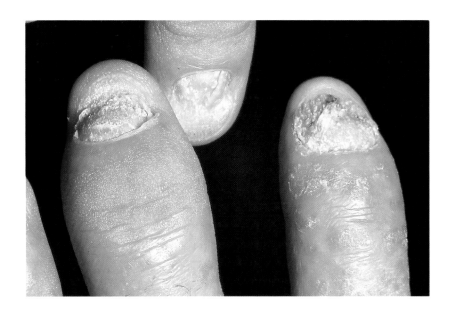

Figure 5.4 Psoriatic nails—fragility associated with arthropathy.

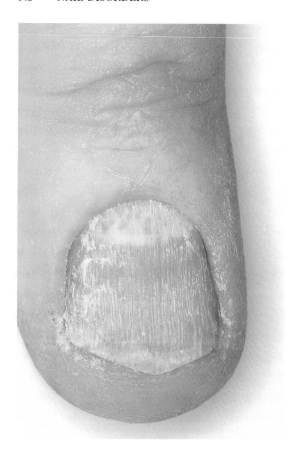

Figure 5.5   Psoriasis—surface 'fine' fragility; trachyonychia appearance.

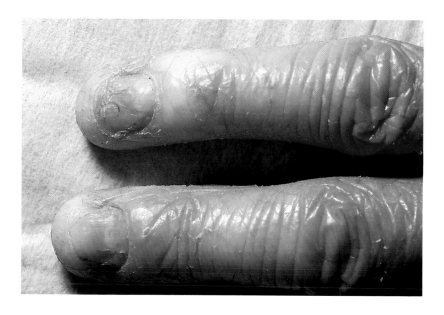

Figure 5.6   Fragile, brittle and soft nails—etretinate treatment.

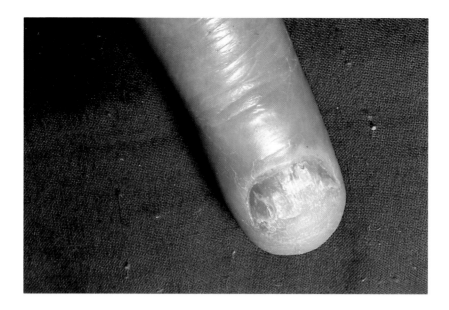

Figure 5.7   Poor (arterial) peripheral circulation nail fragility.

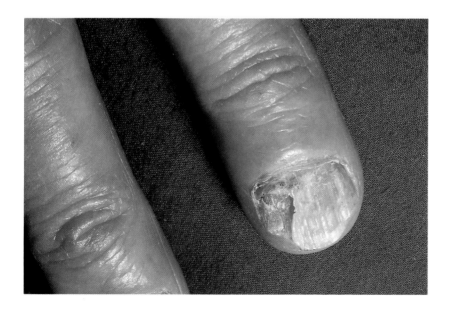

Figure 5.8   Fragile nails in poor (arterial) peripheral circulation.

6

Nail colour changes (Chromonychia)

The term 'chromonychia' indicates an abnormality in colour of the substance, or the surface of the nail plate and/or subungual tissues. Generally, abnormalities of colour depend on the transparency of the nail, its attachments and the character of the underlying tissues. Pigment may accumulate due to overproduction (melanin) or storage (haemosiderin, copper, various drugs); or by surface deposition. The nails provide a historical record—for up to 2 years depending on the rate of linear nail growth—of profound temporary abnormalities of the control of skin pigment which otherwise might pass unnoticed. Colour is also affected by the state of the skin vessels, and various intravascular factors such as anaemia and carbon monoxide poisoning.

Certain important points concerning the examination of abnormal nails are worthy of mention. They should be studied with the subject's fingers completely relaxed and not pressed against any surface. Failure to do this may alter the haemodynamics of the nail and change its appearance. The fingertip should then be blanched to see if the pigmented abnormality is grossly altered; this may help to differentiate between discoloration of the nail plate and of the vascular bed. If the discoloration is in the vascular bed, it will usually disappear. Further information may be gleaned by transillumination of the nail using a pentorch placed against the pulp. If the discoloration is in the matrix or soft tissue, the exact position can more easily be identified. Furthermore, if a topical agent is suspected as the cause, one can remove the discoloration by scrapping or cleaning the nail plate with a solvent such as acetone. If the substance is impregnated more deeply into the nail or subungually, microscopic studies of potassium hydroxide preparations or biopsy specimens using special stains may be indicated. Wood's lamp examination is sometimes useful.

When there is nail contact with occupationally derived agents, or topical application of therapeutic agents, the discoloration often follows the shape of the proximal nail fold. If the discoloration corresponds to the shape of the lunula an internal cause is likely.

Leukonychia (White nail) (Figures 6.1–6.10)

White nails are the most common colour change seen. These can be divided into two main types: 1) true leukonychia, in which the nail plate is involved; 2) apparent leukonychia with involvement of the subungual tissue.

In true leukonychia (Figure 6.1) the nail appears opaque and white in colour owing to the diffraction of light in the abnormal keratotic cells; with polarized light, the nail structure appears disrupted due to disorganization of the keratin fibrils. The leukonychia may be complete, total leukonychia (rare), or incomplete, subtotal leukonychia. These forms can be temporary or permanent depending on the aetiology. Partial forms are divided into punctate leukonychia, which is common, striate leukonychia, relatively common, and distal leukonychia, which is very rare. The term 'pseudoleukonychia' is used when fungal infection involves the nail plate, as, for example, the superficial white onychomycoses, or when nail varnish produces keratin granulation. Apparent leukonychia can be further subdivided into a white appearance of the nail due to: 1) underlying onycholysis and subungual hyperkeratosis; 2) modification of the matrix and/or the nail bed, giving rise, for example, to an apparent macrolunula.

True leukonychia

Total leukonychia (Figure 6.1)

In this rare condition the nail may be milky, chalky, bluish, ivory or porcelain white in colour. The opacity of the whiteness varies: when it is faintly opaque, it may be possible to see transverse streaks of leukonychia in a nail with total leukonychia.

Accelerated nail growth may be associated with total leukonychia.

Subtotal leukonychia

In this form, there is a pink arc of about 2–4 mm width distal to the white area. This can be explained by the fact that the nucleated cells in the distal area mature, lose their keratohyalin granules and then produce healthy keratin several weeks after they have been formed. It is possible that there are parakeratotic cells along the whole length of the nail; these decrease in number as they approach the distal end, thus producing the normal pink colour up to the point of separation from the nail bed. There might, however, be enough left for the nail to acquire a whitish tint when it has lost contact with the nail bed. Some authorities feel that subtotal leukonychia is a phase of total leukonychia based on the occurrence of both in different members of one family and the simultaneous occurrence in one person. In addition, either type may be found separately in some individuals at different times.

Striate leukonychia (Figure 6.4)

One or several nails exhibit a band, usually transverse, 1 or 2 mm wide and often occurring at the same site in each nail.

Punctate leukonychia

In this type, white spots of 1–3 mm in diameter occur singly or in groups; only rarely do they occur on toe nails. Their appearance is usually due to repeated, minor trauma to the matrix. The evolution of the spots is variable; appearing generally on contact with the cuticle, they grow distally with the nail but about half of them disappear in the course of their migration towards the free edge. This proves that parakeratotic cells are capable of maturing and losing their keratohyalin granules to produce keratin, even though they have been without vascularization for many months. Some white spots enlarge, whilst others appear at a distance from the lunula, suggesting that the nail bed is participating by incorporating groups of nucleated cells into the nail. A similar process could explain the exclusively distal leukonychia which is occasionally seen. A local or general fault in keratinization is not the only cause of punctate leukonychia; infiltration of air, which is known to occur in cutaneous parakeratoses, may also play a part.

Leukonychia variegata

This consists of white irregular transverse thread-like streaks.

Longitudinal leukonychia (Figure 6.5)

Longitudinal leukonychia is a typical example of a localized metaplasia. It is characterized by a permanent greyish white longitudinal streak, 1 mm broad, below the nail plate. Histologically there is a mound of horny cells causing the white discoloration due to a lack of transparency resulting in alteration in light diffraction.

Apparent leukonychia

White opacity of the nails in patients with cirrhosis is often known as Terry's nail (Figure 6.6). In the majority of cases, the nails are of an opaque white colour, obscuring the lunula. This discoloration which stops suddenly, 1–2 mm from the distal edge of the nail, leaves a pink area corresponding to the onychodermal band. It lies parallel to the distal part of the nail bed and may be irregular. The condition involves all nails uniformly.

A variation of Terry's nail is the Morey and Burke type in which the whitening of the nail is extended to the central segment with a curved frontal edge. Muehrcke's bands (Figures 6.7, 6.8), which are parallel to the lunula, are separated from one another, and from the lunula, by strips of pink nail. They disappear when the serum albumin level returns to normal and reappear if it falls again. It is possible that hypoalbuminaemia produces oedema of the connective tissue in front of the lunula just below the epidermis of the nail bed, changing the compact arrangement of the collagen in this area into a looser texture, resembling the structure of the lunula; hence the whitish colour. The correlation between the presence or disappearance of the white bands, and the amount of serum albumin, seems to confirm this hypothesis. However, white fingernails preceded by multiple transverse white bands have been reported with normal serum albumin levels.

The ureamic half-and-half nail of Lindsay consists of two parts separated more or less transversely by a well-defined line; the proximal area is dull white, resembling ground glass and obscuring the lunula; the distal area is pink, reddish or brown, and occupies between 20 and 60 per cent of the total length of the nail (average 33 per cent). In typical cases the diagnosis presents no difficulty, but in Terry's nail the pink, distal area may occupy up to 50 per cent of the length of the nail, in which case the two types of nail may be confused. Half-and-half nail can display a normal proximal half portion and the colour of the distal part can be due to either an increase in the number of capillaries and thickening of their walls, or melanic granules in the nail bed. Sometimes the distinctly abnormal onychodermal band extends approximately 20 to 25 per cent from the distal portion of the finger nail as a distal crescent of pigmentation with pigment throughout the brown arc of the nail plate.

Nail changes similar to those reported by Terry, Lindsay and Muehrcke have been termed 'Neapolitan nails'; they are probably simply an age-related phenomenon in otherwise normal individuals.

Anaemia may produce pallor of the nail (apparent leukonychia) if the haemaglobin level falls sufficiently—similar to mucous membrane and conjunctival pallor.

Dermatoses causing leukonychia

In psoriasis the nail may be affected by true leukonychia, due to involvement of the matrix, and apparent leukonychia, due to onycholysis;

and by parakeratosis deposits in the nail bed. One of the earliest signs of leprosy is an apparent macrolunula, which may become total in dystrophic leprosy. Leukonychia may also occur in other dermatoses, such as alopecia areata, dyshidrosis and Darier's disease (Figure 6.9).

The box on page 149 shows a comprehensive list of many causes and factors leading to leukonychia.

Some causes of leukonychia

Congenital and/or hereditary	Isolated Acrokeratosis verruciformis (Hopf) Associated with koilonychia—LEOPARD syndrome (lentigines, electrocardiographic changes, ocular hypertelorism, pulmonary stenosis, abnormalities of genitalia, retarded growth, deafness) Associated with deafness Leukonychia totalis, multiple sebaceous cysts, renal calculi Darier's disease—usually linear and longitudinal Psoriasis
Acquired	
Pseudoleukonychia	Diffuse form of distal and lateral subungual onychomycosis Superficial white onychomycosis Keratin granulation (superficial friability from nail varnish)
Apparent leukonychia	Anaemia Cancer chemotherapeutic agents Cirrhosis (Terry's sign) Dyshidrosis Half-and-half nail (renal diseases) and distal crescent pigmentation Leprosy Muehrcke's lines of hypoalbuminaemia
True leukonychia	Alkaline metabolic disease Alopecia areata Carcinoid tumours of the bronchus Cardiac insufficiency Cytotoxic and other drugs (emetine, pilocarpine, sulphonamide, cortisone) Erythema multiforme Exfoliative dermatitis Fasting periods in orthodox Jews and Moslems Fracture Gout Hodgkin's disease Hypocalcaemia Infectious diseases and infectious fevers Intra-abdominal malignancies Kidney transplant Leuko-onycholysis paradentotica Leprosy Menstrual cycle Myocardial infarction Occupational Pellagra Peripheral neuropathy Poisoning (antimony, arsenic, fluoride, lead, thallium) Protein deficiency Psychotic episodes (acute) Renal failure (acute or chronic) Shock Sickle cell anaemia Surgery Sympathetic leukonychia Trauma Tumours (benign), cysts pressing on matrix Ulcerative colitis Zinc deficiency

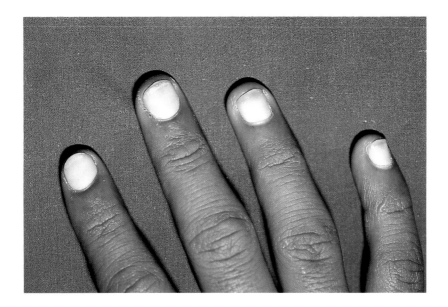

Figure 6.1   Total (true) leukonychia—congenital; all 20 nails affected in this individual.

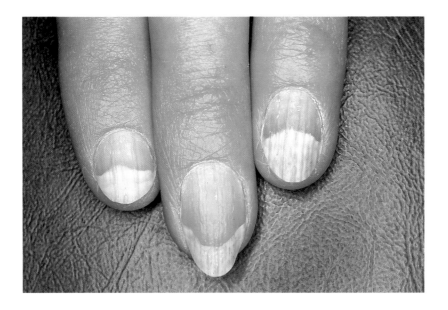

Figure 6.2   Apparent leukonychia due to onycholysis (due to hyperthyroidism in this individual).

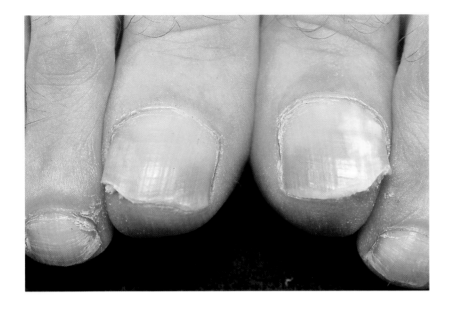

Figure 6.3   Pseudoleukonychia due to onychomycosis.

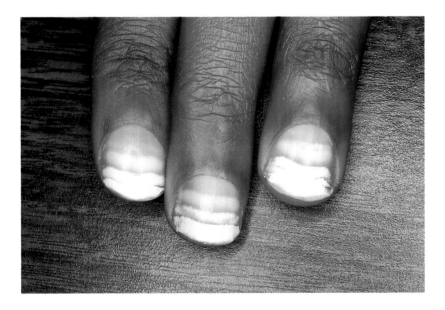

Figure 6.4   Striate (true) leukonychia—congenital.

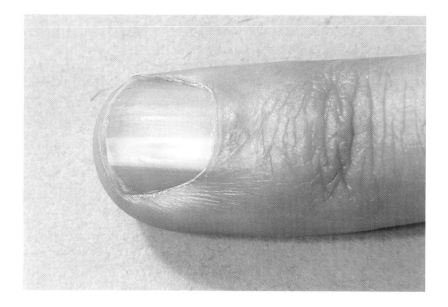

Figure 6.5   Longitudinal true leukonychia, in this case congenital; but if acquired and single may be due to proximal benign tumour or cyst impairing keratinization.

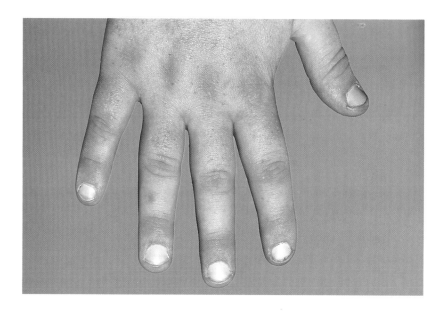

Figure 6.6   Apparent leukonychia associated with liver disease (acquired) and anaemia.

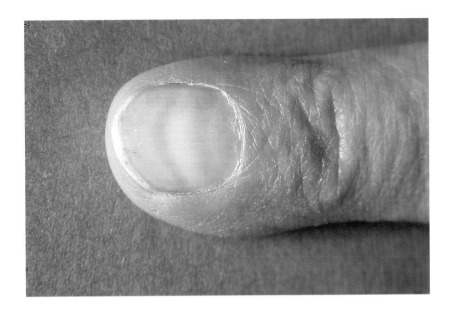

Figure 6.7   Banded apparent leukonychia due to hypoalbuminaemia (Muehrcke's band).

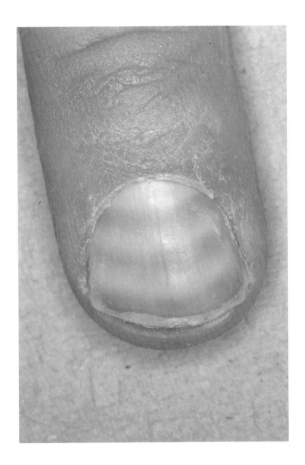

Figure 6.8   Apparent leukonychia (double Muehrcke's band).

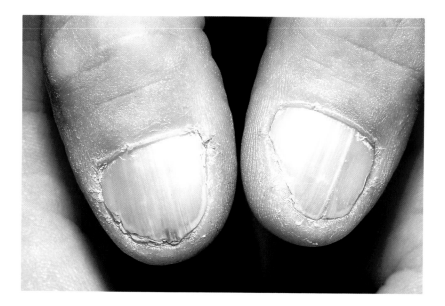

Figure 6.9   Longitudinal white lines of Darier's disease.

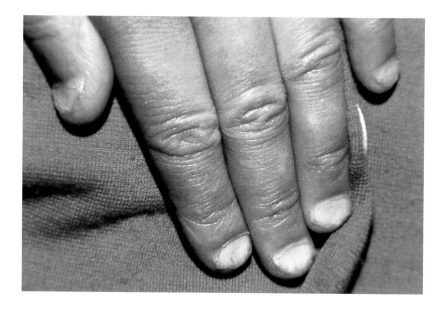

Figure 6.10   True leukonychia with koilonychia—may be associated with deafness.

Melanonychia (Brown/Black nail) (Figures 6.11–6.15)

This colour change is potentially the most serious because malignant melanoma (see Chapter 4) may present in many guises—but many less significant abnormalities can produce brown or black discoloration (see box). Most of the causes will be self-evident at the time of presentation either from the history or on careful medical examination.

Some causes of melanonychia

Black	Naevi
	Racial (Figure 4.29)
	Drugs, eg adriamycin, cyclophosphamide
	Haemorrhage (Figures 6.11, 6.12)
	Malignant melanoma (Figures 4.30, 4.32–34, 4.36)
	Onychomycoses—saprophytic
Brown	Exogenous
	Drugs and dyes, eg dithranol, potassium permanganate, silver nitrate (Figures 6.13, 6.14)
	Endogenous
	Naevi
	Racial—negroid and mongoloid
	Addison's disease (Figure 6.15)
	Drugs, eg chlorpromazine, tetracyclines, ketoconazole, sulphonamides, cytotoxics, acyclovir
	Fetal hydantoin syndrome
	Haemochromatosis
	Laugier–Hunziker syndrome (Figure 4.30)
	Malnutrition
	Nail enamels and hardeners
	Peutz–Jeghers syndrome
	Pregnancy
	Thyroid disease

In clinical practice the main type presenting to the dermatologist is the brown or black line on the nail—longitudinal linear melanonychia (LM) and its sequelae; the linear band may be in the nail plate and the nail bed (Figures 4.29, 4.30, 6.15). Despite our increased knowledge of the subject, the appearance of longitudinal melanonychia still perplexes the physician and distresses the patient. The cause of medical concern stems from the similarity in appearance of benign longitudinal melanonychia and malignant melanoma. The nail plate is derived from an invagination, the ungual cul-de-sac, containing the nail matrix. The proximal part of the matrix produces the superficial third portion of the nail plate, and the other portion of the matrix produces the rest. The changes observed in the nail plate often reflect what is taking place in the matrix. The band of excess melanin is due to a localized increase in the number and/or function of normal or abnormal melanocytes in the matrix, and its linear pattern is due to the unique growth dynamics of the nail plate. Since longitudinal melanonychia represents a focus of melanocytic activity in the matrix it is possible to identify which portion of the matrix is involved by determining the level of the melanin pigment revealed in transverse histological sections of the nail plate. It is now well established that functional melanocytes are present in the normal nail matrix, having migrated during the 16th to the 17th week of gestation. The melanocytes in the distal portion of the nail matrix are more numerous ($300/mm^2$) and more strongly dihydroxyphenylalanine (dopa) positive than are those in the proximal portion. This explains why most of the pigmented lesions of nails arise distally, making surgical intervention easier to carry out with few adverse sequelae likely; in contrast to operations involving the proximal matrix which often cause nail dystrophy with obvious scarring. These melanocytes differ from those at other sites in the skin; they are fewer and are present in the lower two to four cell layers, rather than being confined to the basal layer. They are normally non-functional: when they are activated, melanosomes are transferred via dendrites to the cornified matrix cells as they grow outward to form the nail plate. All stages of melanosomal development have been demonstrated by electron microscopy in subungual melanocytes.

Longitudinal melanonychia is normal in all deeply pigmented races. In Negroes and Orientals, melanocytes are much more abundant in the matrix than in Caucausians. Almost 100 per cent of Negroes have longitudinal melanonychia as a normal feature. Approximately 11 per cent of normal Japanese subjects have pigmented bands on the nails. In sharp contrast, longitudinal melanonychia is unusual in white Caucasians. Since longitudinal melanonychia may be one of the earliest manifestations of malignant melanoma, it is important to note that subungual malignant melanoma occurs in 2–3 per cent of malignant melanoma in white Caucasians, as well as in Japanese, but in 15 to 20 per cent of malignant melanoma in Negroes. The incidence of melanoma in the nail region is, however, little different between these racial groups since blacks rarely present with malignant melanoma affecting other sites (interestingly, 31 per cent of subungual melanomas begin as a linear streak in Japanese cases).

Bearing in mind the potential risk of malignant melanoma, one should rule out the other conditions that may present with this sign (see box). When no specific cause is found, the following features should be considered regarding possible malignant melanoma:

● Extension of the linear pigmentation to the free edge of the nail

● Only one finger affected

● Periungual spread of the pigmentation

● Darkening of the band

● Progressive widening of the linear streak with blurring of its border

● Age over 50 years.

One should also rule out the following:

● Periungual pigmented areas in Laugier–Hunziker syndrome (benign)

Some causes of longitudinal melanonychia

Idiopathic

Racial
  Dark-skinned races (negroid and mongoloid)

Systemic
  Addison's disease of the adrenal gland
  Adrenalectomy for Cushing's disease
  Carcinoma of the breast
  Drugs
  Irradiation
  Malnutrition
  Photochemotherapy
  Pregnancy
  Secondary syphilis
  Vitamin B12 deficiency

Dermatological
  Amyloid (primary)
  Basal cell carcinoma
  Bacterial infection
  Bowen's disease
  Fungal infection
  Laugier–Hunziker syndrome
  Lichen planus
  Malignant melanoma
  Peutz–Jeghers–Touraine syndrome
  Porphyria cutanea tarda
  Radiotherapy and radiodermatitis

Regional and local
  Carpal tunnel syndrome
  Repeated minor injuries
  Trauma (acute)

● Single LM due to metastases of distant malignant melanoma

● Non-migratory haematoma or foreign body.

The dangers of misdiagnosis are:
a) that the proper treatment of a subungual melanoma will be delayed, and the tumour will grow and disseminate.
b) that treatment as for subungual melanoma will lead to over-treatment of a benign lesion; and thus to unnecessary surgery. Therefore excisional biopsy is crucial.

What can be expected from histological examination? Lesions within the matrix that produces LM can be roughly divided into subungual melanosis and melanoma in situ. The first group includes:

a) Secondary stimulation of non-functioning melanocytes as may occur with trauma, etc.

b) Increased numbers and activity of normal-appearing melanocytes resulting in single or multiple longitudinal bands of the type which is common in dark-skinned races, as well as in 1 per cent of white-skinned. Also included in this group are lentigo simplex and melanocytic naevus.

It must be emphasized that this group of 'benign hyperplasias' represents a histological spectrum ranging from increased production of melanin with normal numbers of melanocytes at one end, to both increased production of melanin and increased number of cells at the other. The lentigo, characterized by elongated rete ridges and a corresponding increased number of functional melanocytes in the basal layer, occupies a middle position in the spectrum. Nests of melanocytes sometimes appear at the dermal–epidermal junctioin suggesting possible instability or early malignancy.

In melanoma in situ there are increased numbers of atypical melanocytes. Acral lentiginous melanoma in situ exhibits atypical melanocytes in all layers of the matrix epithelium and also in the dermis of the matrix acral.

The problem of recurrent LM following surgical removal has not yet been studied in contrast to the recurrent pigmentation following partial or total excision of some pigmented lesions such as melanocytic naevi or malignant melanoma at other sites.

One should therefore ask: Was the original histological interpretation correct? Is the recurrent process still identical or different? How can one prevent recurrences?

So far there are no proven examples of a benign melanocytic process becoming malignant due to the biopsy of recurrent LM; but after a third recurrence the authors have found a melanocytic naevus which was not diagnosed histologically in two previous biopsies.

The suggested guidelines, using different procedures, should at least partially preclude the relapsing of nail pigmentation. The following guidelines should be adhered to where possible to enable accurate tissue diagnosis to be made and appropriate treatment carried out.

As a first step, the anatomical site of the matrix affected will be obtained from the level of the melanin pigment identified with Fontana's silver stain of a nail clipping obtained from the distal free edge. The type of biopsy selected will then depend on:

● the site of the matrix melanin production linked with

● the width of the linear pigmentation

● the site of the band in the nail plate.

If the pigment is located within the ventral portion of the nail plate, a decision has to be made depending on the width of the band:

a) A punch biopsy should be used when the width of the band is less than 3 mm. Removal of the base of the nail plate allows one to release the specimen in an easier manner, and above all to check the integrity of the region, distal to the biopsied matrix area.

b) A transverse matrix biopsy for a band wider than 3 mm.

If the pigment involves the upper portion of the nail, it is obviously difficult to use the two previous procedures to remove the source of melanin pigment, for anatomical reasons and because of the risk of a secondary dystrophy:

c) A rectangular block of tissue is therefore excised using two parallel incisions down to the bone. An L-shaped incision is carried back along the lateral nail wall freeing this flap. The lateral section may then be rotated medially and approximated to the remaining nail segment, or

d) If the band is wider than 6 mm or if the whole thickness of the nail is involved by the pigment, surgical removal of the nail apparatus seems the most logical method. However, one (or even two) 3 mm punch biopsy could be an alternative before more radical treatment is undertaken, especially in young women.

When the band lies within the lateral third of the nail plate, lateral-longitudinal biopsy is more suitable.

e) If LM is accompanied by periungual pigmentation (Hutchinson's sign), removal of the nail apparatus is required.

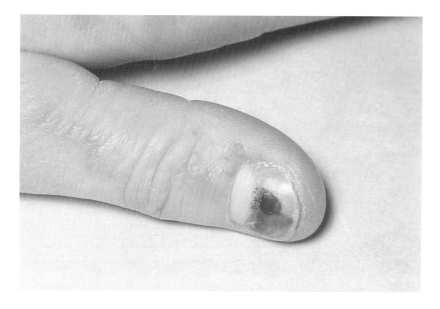

Figure 6.11   Nail bed black stain due to traumatic haemorrhage.

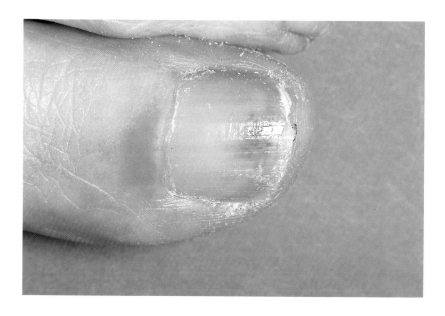

Figure 6.12   Focal black area due to subungual haemorrhage—trauma.

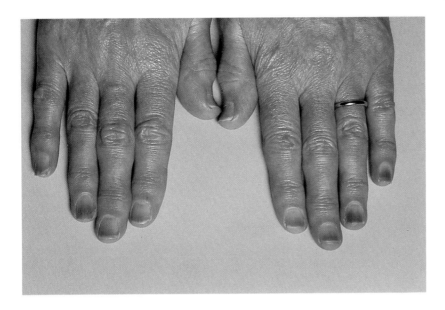

Figure 6.13 Brown stain of all finger nails—exogenous due to henna dye.

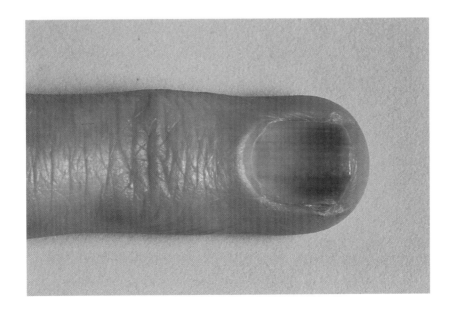

Figure 6.14 Magnified view of one digit as in Figure 6.13; henna staining.

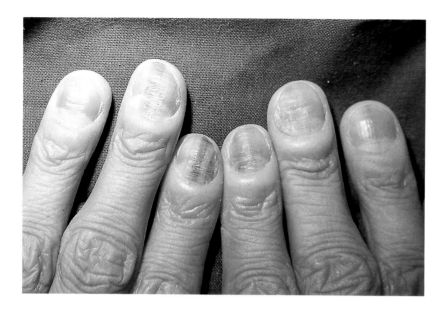

Figure 6.15 Multiple longitudinal melanonychia in Addison's disease—hypoadrenalism. Mild chronic paronychia (*Candida type*) also present.

Other discolorations (Figures 6.16–6.22)

The variety of colour changes that may occur in the nail apparatus, other than white and brown-black, are listed in the following box. Many are due to obvious cosmetic procedures, topical or oral drugs, or common diseases. None is of particular significance in itself, its presence sometimes aiding in the diagnosis of disease or pointing towards overdose of drugs.

Some causes of discolorations

Yellow	Yellow nail syndromes (Figures 6.17–6.18) Nail enamel and hardeners AIDS Carotene Dermatophyte onychomycosis (Figure 6.16) Drugs—tetracycline (fluorescent lunula), penicillamine. clioquinole (topical), mepacrine (nail bed) Jaundice
Blue/blue-grey	Antimalarials Argyria Bleomycin Congenital pernicious anaemia Minocycline Phenolphthalein Phenothiazines Wilson's disease
Green	*Aspergillus* Bullous disorders Jaundice 'Old' haematoma (green-yellow) *Pseudomonas aeruginosa* (Figure 6.20)

Red/purple	Angioma
	Cirsoid aneurysm tumour
	Glomus tumour (Figure 7.5)
	Congestive cardiac failure (lunula)
	Enchondroma
	Heparin (transverse)
	Lichen planus
	Linear red line
	   Darier's disease
	   Benign tumours/cysts near proximal matrix
	Lupus erythematosus
	Porphyria (with fluorescent light)
	Rheumatoid arthritis
	Warfarin

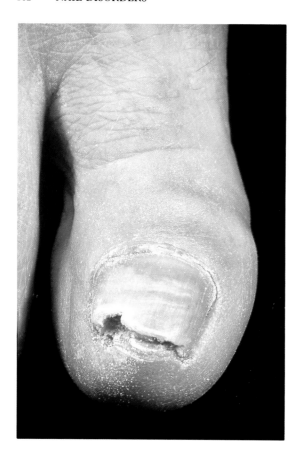

Figure 6.16   Yellow nail—onychomycosis.

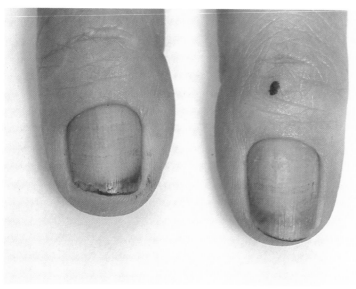

Figure 6.17   Transverse overcurvature and vague yellowing in yellow nail syndrome (early stage).

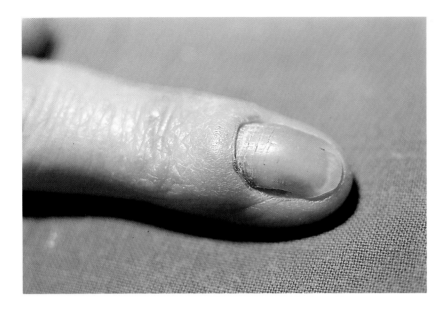

Figure 6.18   Yellow nail syndrome.

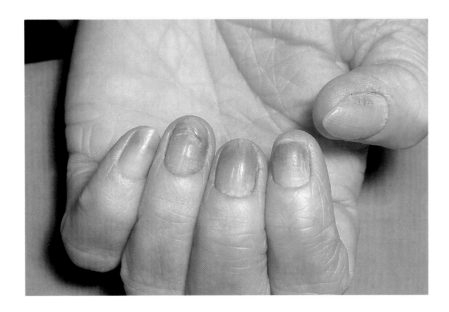

Figure 6.19   Yellow nail syndrome—established yellow colour in all nails.

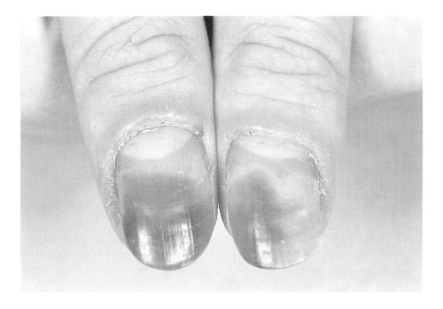

Figure 6.20   Green/yellow discoloration—onycholysis and *Pseudomonas pyocyanea* staining.

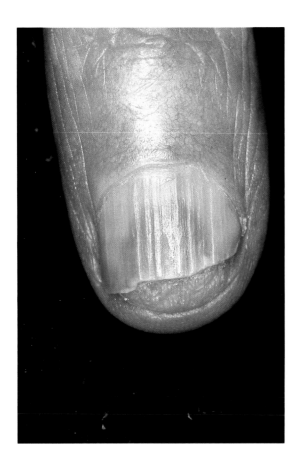

Figure 6.21   Reddish nail bed colour due to psoriasis.

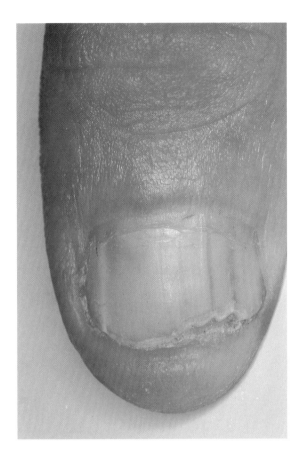

Figure 6.22   Longitudinal red lines in Darier's disease plus associated white lines.

Further reading

Melanonychia

Baran R and **Kechijian P,** Longitudinal melanonychia (melanonychia striata): diagnosis and management. *J Am Acad Dermatol* (1989) **21**:1165–75.

Other discolorations

Daniel CR III, Nail pigmentation abnormalities. *Dermatol Clin* (1985) **3**:431–43.

7
The painful nail

(Figures 7.1–7.6)

Pain is a non-specific and common symptom of many conditions of the nail apparatus (see box on page 168). Apart from various forms of trauma, many inflammatory and vascular diseases may cause pain; however, pain is so subjective and inconstant a symptom that even diseases commonly known as being particularly painful may follow a rather asymptomatic course and vice versa. The entire distal phalanx, especially the finger pulp, is richly innervated. Each space-occupying process, whether inflammatory or neoplastic, may produce pain because the subungual tissue consists of dense fibrous tissue closely adherent to the bone and without the 'elastic' pad of subcutaneous fat. Inflammatory conditions and tumours are squeezed in this firm subungual tissue between

the hard nail plate and hard bone, although slowly enlarging processes may lead to clubbing and pressure-induced bone erosion. Pain is therefore to be expected under these conditions. In addition, the tumour itself may be inherently painful, a point well-illustrated by the glomus tumour. If pain subsequent to simple trauma or acute inflammation does not respond to adequate therapy, either an X-ray or biopsy or both should be performed to rule out a malignant tumour. X-rays may be difficult to interpret, especially in the elderly with degenerative arthritis, and it may be necessary to repeat the X-rays or other imaging techniques if the disease does not follow the expected course, or if it fails to respond to treatment.

Some causes of painful nail

Trauma	Splinters/foreign bodies Crush and squeeze injuries (Figure 7.1) Sportsman, sports shoe injuries Cold injury Ingrowing toe nail Childhood malalignment (Figure 7.2) Common type (Figure 7.3)
Inflammation	Acute (and chronic) paronychia Subcutaneous abscess Subungual foreign body Prosector's wart (Tb) Osteomyelitis Herpes simplex Postcryosurgery—may be prolonged bone pain Ventral pterygium Dorsolateral fissures Pincer nail—severe form enclosing bone (Figure 7.4) Acroosteolysis Implantation epidermoid cyst Sarcoid dactylitis
Tumours (soft tissue and bone)	Glomus tumour (Figure 7.5) Subungual wart Subungual corn Subungual papilloma—incontinentia pigmenti Keratoacanthoma Bowen's disease Squamous cell carcinoma Secondary infection—slow-growing tumours Leiomyoma Some neuromas Fibroma Osteoma, exostosis Enchondroma (Figure 7.6) Osteoid osteoma Aneurysmal bone cyst Myxoid cyst
Vascular	Chilblains Raynaud's phenomenon/disease Systemic sclerosis Rheumatoid vasculitic lesions

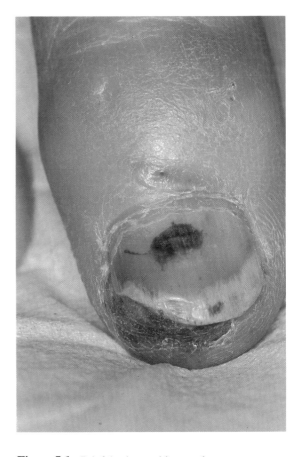

Figure 7.1 Painful subungual haemorrhage.

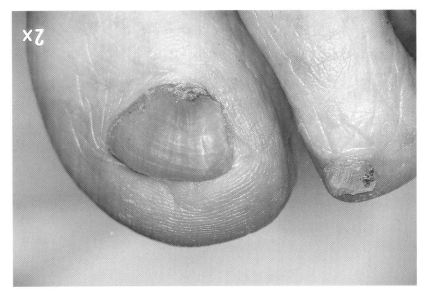

(a)

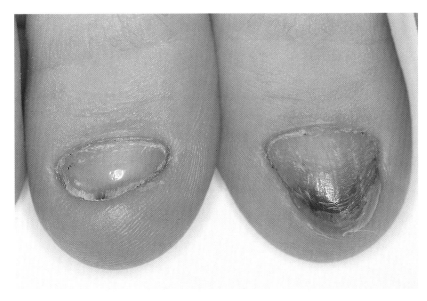

(b)

Figure 7.2 (a) Onychogryphosis produces pain by pressure on the lateral nail wall. (b) Congenital malalignment of great toe nails—may ingrow and be painful, particularly with crawling.

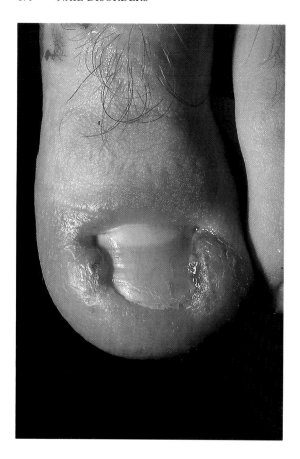

Figure 7.3   Painful inflamed ingrowing great toe nail.

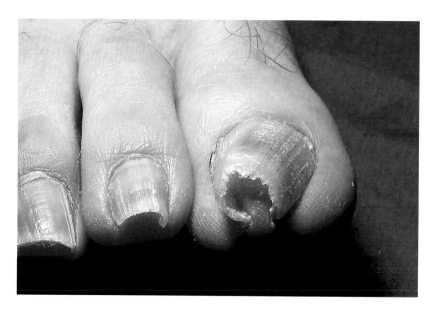

Figure 7.4   Toe pincer nail deformity—may be painful, particularly if bone is affected.

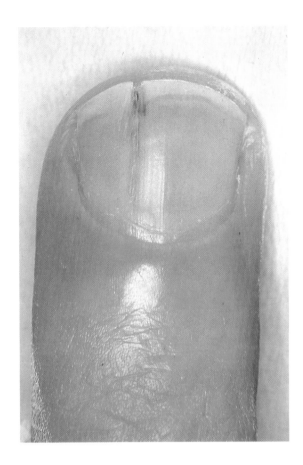

Figure 7.5 Glomus tumour—usually painful despite minimal signs.

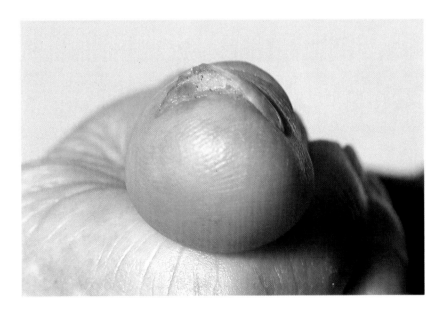

Figure 7.6 Nail dystrophy due to painful subungual enchondroma.

8

Treatment of common nail disorders

Psoriasis

Despite many recent advances in the treatment of psoriasis in general, the management of nail psoriasis is tedious and unsatisfactory for patient and physician—indeed many doctors justify a *laissez-faire* stance because of poor therapeutic success rates and the inconvenience or side-effects noted by the patient. The following may be of use in selected cases:

1. *Photochemotherapy*. This will produce benefit in some cases within 6 months—for patients with severe nail involvement it may be fully justifiable to continue treatment long after the skin psoriasis has totally cleared. It is difficult to decide whether to use high-intensity UVA just to the affected nails individually, after either topical or oral psoralens; or oral psoralen with total-body PUVA, the latter on the basis that systemic as well as local factors are important in clearing psoriasis. However, even doses of UVA 2.5–5 times that which are needed to clear psoriasis on glabrous skin have shown only limited success. Side-effects include subungual haemorrhage, photo-onycholysis and pigmentation of the nail—even longitudinal melanonychia.

2. *Oral retinoids*. In general, the results of etretinate therapy have been poor for most common types of nail psoriasis—partly because of the limited efficacy of the drug and because doses

in the higher therapeutic range may cause fragility or atrophy of any newly formed nail. Therefore good results will pertain to psoriasis with thick nails.

Acropustulosis and the pustular nail changes of common peripheral pustular psoriasis respond in some degree in the short term but relapse is common within 1 to 3 months of stopping treatment. Combined etretinate/PUVA treatment is said to lower the frequency of relapse.

The principal metabolite of etretinate acitrenin has identical efficacy and side-efffects.

3. *Topical treatments*. Limited success has been obtained using 1 per cent fluorouracil solution dissolved in propylene glycol applied twice daily for approximately 6 months around the nail margins—it has only been recommended in the presence of pitting and hypertrophy and not in the onycholytic type.

Potent topical steroids are widely prescribed but probably only function well in suppressing inflammatory types of nail apparatus psoriasis. Clobetasol propionate cream, with or without plastic occlusive dressings, is the most effective for short-term use. To aid penetration topical steroids have been used combined with 5–10 per cent benzoyl peroxide, 0.1 per cent retinoic acid cream, or 2–5 per cent salicylic acid.

Intralesional jet injections of corticosteroids, widely used many years ago, have fallen into disuse because of difficulties in sterilizing the equipment against viral contamination (hepatitis and HIV in particular)—but also because of rapid relapse after initial improvement.

4. *Systemic treatment*. Methotrexate has not been generally recommended for the treatment of psoriasis limited to the nail apparatus. However, the crippling effects of severe pustular nail dystrophies justify this in practice: anecdotal reports suggest some benefit in doses of 10–20 mg oral methotrexate weekly—for 12–18 months minimum time. When methotrexate is used for recalcitrant psoriasis vulgaris, the associated common nail changes only improve slowly since the drug slows nail growth rates by up to 100 per cent less than the normal rates, so that even fingernail psoriasis may take longer than 2 years to clear.

The antimitotic drug Razoxane® initially showed great value for psoriasis and any associated arthropathy and nail dystrophy; it has now been withdrawn from general use since leukaemia occurred in many of those taking the treatment.

5. *X-irradiation*. Once widely used, this mode of treatment is now reserved for selected recalcitrant cases. Superficial low-voltage X-ray may be used—total dose per area, per lifetime, should not exceed 10 Gy.

6. *General*. If onycholysis is present, the nail plate should be trimmed back to the point of separation—particularly if local subungual treatment is to be applied with any hope of success. Sometimes chemical avulsion with urea may help in the management of hypertrophic nail psoriasis.

Secondary invasion by *Candida* species, moulds or *Pseudomonas* is common and should be treated with a topical imidazole cream or antiseptic as appropriate.

Unfortunately, whatever the treatment used, failure and recurrence are common. Concealing 'flat' dystrophies with nail varnish may be valuable and in hypertrophic forms a chiropodist or podiatrist may be of great help.

Lichen planus

Treatment of lichen planus of the nail apparatus is entirely symptomatic, the results ultimately depending on the type treated and its overall prognosis, for example, early scarring and erosive types respond worst of all.

Some general principles regarding management and treatment can be stated:

a) If the nails are mildly affected, for example with single depressions, or the longitudinal melanonychia type, treatment is of no help.

b) If ridging is prominent with thinning and fragility then oral or intralesional steroids may help—Prednisolone 60 mg daily for 4 to 6 weeks followed by reduction of the dose to 20 mg daily for up to 1 year. As an alternative, triamcinolone acetonide may be injected intramuscularly (80 mg the first month, then 40 mg monthly for 6 months). The frequency of the injections should be adjusted to the patient's response. Treatment may last for 18 months to 9 years. Intralesional triamcinolone (or hydrocortisone) injected into the nail matrix (0.5 ml per digit per treatment) monthly for 6 months, then at 3–6 month intervals, is used in many centres and good initial results can be obtained. It is, however, painful and requires a patient of great fortitude.

c) Scarring and atrophic varieties may be temporarily arrested by the above treatments.

d) Patients with painful ulcerative lichen planus may get symptomatic relief from twice-daily application of clobetasol propionate cream; failing this, skin grafting may help.

e) When a 'twenty nail dystrophy' shows histological evidence of lichen planus, no treatment is required since the prognosis is good.

f) In patients for whom systemic steroids are contra-indicated, oral etretinate or acitretin can be considered in view of their (limited) success in lichen planus of the skin and oral mucous membrane—the difficulty is in 'titrating' the dose to produce benefit without side-effects. The highest standard doses may cause nail fragility, atrophy and periungual granulation tissue.

Onychomycosis

There are many drugs that can satisfactorily kill onychomycotic fungi under laboratory conditions in vitro. In clinical practice there is difficulty in obtaining high cure rates because of the slow response to treatment, poor patient compliance, failure of adequate penetration of topically applied agents and the slowness of incorporation of systemic drugs into the affected nail. Only rarely is fungal drug resistance a significant problem. Prior to commencing treatment one must ask whether therapy is necessary—after due explanation of the limitations of treatment, many asymptomatic patients will be satisfied to 'leave well alone'.

To ensure that any treatment carried out may be given correctly, the following factors should be taken into consideration:

1. The type of onychomycosis including the site of involvement and the identity of the organism.
2. The rate of linear growth of the toe nails, which is one-third to one-half that of finger nails.

Fungi gain entry into the nail by three main routes, resulting in different clinical patterns of infection:

1. From the distal subungual area and the lateral nail groove giving rise to distal and lateral subungual onychomycosis (DLSO);
2. The dorsal aspect of the nail plate as superficial white onychomycosis (SWO);
3. The undersurface of the proximal nail fold.

This yields two types:

a) Primary. The organism invades the undersurface of the nail giving rise to proximal white subungual onychomycosis (PWSO).
b) Secondary to chronic paronychia where the nail can be affected at one or both lateral surfaces.

Total dystrophic onychomycosis may result from the progression of any of the previously mentioned forms of infection or it may appear primarily in chronic mucocutaneous candidosis (CMCC).

Isolation of fungi

Whatever the method of treatment chosen, confirmation of the diagnosis is vital before commencement, since all forms of therapy are prolonged and the futility of long-term antifungal therapy in the absence of any fungus is obvious.

Despite the characteristic appearance in potassium hydroxide preparations, *Scopulariopsis brevicaulis* or *Hendersonula toruloidea*, culture of fungus is indispensable. It is sometimes difficult to isolate fungi in culture, even from nails positive on direct microscopy. The problem is compounded if the patient has already received topical or systemic treatment; or if the hyphae in the most accessible part of the nail plate are not viable.

How can one determine whether a cultured fungus is a commensal or truly responsible for the nail dystrophy? According to many major authorities the criteria for the diagnosis of onychomycosis include:

● If a dermatophyte is isolated it is taken to be the pathogen without supporting evidence.

● If a mould or yeast is isolated, it is only considered of significance if the appropriate fungal elements (mycelium, arthrospores or yeast cells) are seen in direct microscopy of the nails.

● For a diagnosis of mould infection, no dermatophyte must have been isolated on actidione-containing or actidione-free medium, and at least 5/20 inocula must have yielded the mould.

These criteria are controversial: dermatophytes, known as primary nail pathogens, may follow the development of onycholysis due to repeated minor trauma of the great toe nail. By contrast, *Scopulariopsis brevicaulis* has features of both primary and secondary nail pathogens and can be found in both previously healthy as well as in diseased nails.

Other experts give stress to the importance of histological examination showing the presence of hyphal location of the fungus in nail keratin. This avoids the error of a false-negative culture in dermatophyte infection. This technique also rules out the non-dermatophyte fungi cultured from the nails if they cannot be demonstrated histologically (false-positive cultures).

For early diagnosis of PWSO a 3 mm punch biopsy restricted to the nail and taken from the white area is indispensable, as is culture from this specimen. The hyphae are located in the deeper portion of the nail and the superficial layers of the nail bed.

Why are current treatments unsatisfactory?

Topical therapy alone is only effective in SWO which is usually produced by *Tricophyton mentagrophytes interdigitale* and sometimes by non-dermatophyte moulds such as *Cephalosporium*, *Aspergillus* species and *Fusarium*. Superficial abrasion followed by azoles (lotions or creams) or 10 per cent glutaraldehyde solution may be used.

Chronic paronychia with *Candida* infection can also benefit from local treatment, such as an imidazole or nystatin combined with topical steroid, providing that the conditions favouring its growth have been eliminated by using cotton gloves lining rubber gloves for 'wet work'.

Nevertheless, there is poor penetration of active compounds despite the appearance of promising chemicals such as 5 per cent ciclopiroxolamine or 28 per cent tioconazole.

Drug-related toxicity may limit the use of oral therapy. Griseofulvin is active against dermatophytes. In general 1 g daily is indicated in adults and 15 mg/kg body weight in children. The drug, being lipophilic, must be taken with food. Minor side-effects such as nausea and headache are common; photosensitivity and systemic lupus erythematosus are very rare.

Ketoconazole has a broad spectrum since it is active against dermatophyte infection and *Candida* species. It is given in a single dose of 200 mg daily with the main meal. Besides minor side-effects such as dizziness, headache and gastro-intestinal intolerance, the drug is weakly anti-

androgenic (gynaecomastia). Therapeutic agents reducing gastric acidity should be taken at least 2 hours after ketoconazole. Hepatotoxicity has been reported (1:10 000 treated cases). Since some deaths have occurred in patients treated for onychomycosis, careful monitoring of liver function at fortnightly intervals is mandatory for 2 months, then at monthly intervals. This drug is now mainly used for severe or systematized fungal infections—for instance immunosuppressed individuals, due to disease or drugs.

Oral antifungal therapy is necessarily prolonged: 6 months for finger nails, 12 to 18 months for the great toe nail; and may be unsuccessful because of poor patient compliance to such prolonged treatment, or inadequate dosage. The systemic antifungal drugs act clinically as a barrier to the invasion of the fungus toward the proximal areas of the nail plate. To test this barrier effect a notch is made with a scalpel and filled with silver nitrate. If an effective drug is given, the onychomycotic area does not invade proximal to the mark. The subject is monitored monthly.

How can one improve the results of treatment?

An adjunct to antifungal chemotherapy should be used in removing as much nail material containing fungi as possible:
a) mechanically by cutting, filing, abrading
b) chemically by keratinolysis (eg urea nail avulsion)
c) surgically by nail avulsion
All these physical and chemical techniques are intended to shorten the duration of treatment but they are also open to some criticisms:

1. Nail plate abrasion is not sufficient, the nail bed still being abnormal.
2. With urea used for nail avulsion, only the clinically affected nail is detachable and fungal organisms may well be present in the margin of the 'normal' adherent portion of the nail; also it is technically difficult, when using the chemical ablation method, to ensure that infected nail

material under the proximal nail fold is completely removed. This explains the better results obtained when using a combined urea/imidazole preparation.

3. After surgical avulsion of the nail, the loss of the counterpressure normally produced by the nail plate allows progressive expansion of the distal soft tissue and the free edge of regrowing nail may then embed itself in the unrestricted growth of the underlying distal nail bed. The use of partial surgical avulsion of the nail is suitable for onychomycosis of limited extent and results in reasonable remission rates while reducing the time needed for systemic therapy.

Treatment of various sub-types

Onychomycosis caused by moulds

a) It is easy to eradicate the moulds responsible for SWO as mentioned above.

b) *Scopulariopsis brevicaulis* or *Pyrenochaeta unguis-hominis* need repeated chemical removal of the nail followed by local applications of keratolytics.

c) *Hendersonula toruloidea* or *Scytalidium hyalinum* infections can be treated by topical 28 per cent tioconazol.

Onychomycosis caused by *Candida*

a) The nail drystrophy can be treated with oral ketoconazole if severe enough or with chemical avulsion followed by local antifungal treatment.

b) In CMCC the dose of ketoconazole may have to be increased to 400 or 600 mg daily.

c) Onycholysis should be treated locally by trimming the nail as far back as possible. The nail bed should be brushed with soap for 2–3 days, then with an imidazole lotion. Wet work should be avoided as much as possible, with two pairs of gloves (cotton under rubber).

d) In chronic paronychia systemic therapy with ketoconazole is no more efficacious than topical treatment. The addition of intralesional steroid injections may be useful. Treatment should not be considered complete until the cuticle has regrown. If foreign bodies are suspected (occupational origin), surgical therapy removing a crescent of swollen proximal nail fold is efficient.

A new area is now opening in the treatment of onychomycosis, providing 1) shortening of curative treatment by all methods (3 months of finger nails, 6 months for toe nails); 2) appearance of new drugs with broad spectrum and good tolerance such as itraconazole, fluconazole and terbinafine; the latter has shown good results in early studies and will shortly be 'competing' with the available oral agents for onychomycosis; 3) preventative local treatment after the cure of onychomycosis around the affected nail, and the toewebs; more topical treatments with good success rates possibly becoming available (eg nail lacquer therapies such as Amorolfine, currently under review).

Periungual warts

Periungual and subungual warts in general last longer than other types of common warts (verruca vulgaris) of the fingers and toes; even when the latter exist in the same individual they tend to have a shorter natural history and remit sooner. The lifespan of periungual warts may be such that they, and the various treatments, may exceed the patience of both patient and physician! Under such circumstances intelligent placebo therapy may well be appropriate.

A great variety of treatments are listed in all pharmacopoeias, reflecting their individually limited success rates.

Treatments

Liquid nitrogen

The use of liquid nitrogen is convenient and efficient, but lesions frozen around the nails may produce throbbing, intense pain, secondary to oedema under the nail bed. One must also be aware that the skin of both infants and the elderly often swells more than might normally be expected in intermediate age groups.

Haemorrhagic bullae may be cosmetically unpleasant but usually painless: they develop within 12–24 hours and remain for about 7–10 days before drying. Their premature rupture does not alter the course of healing. Application of clobetasol propionate before treatment reduces the inflammatory response to the freeze and may be continued twice a day for 2–3 days. Oral aspirin 600 mg, three times daily, commencing 2 hours before, and for 3 days after treatment minimizes pain.

Monochloracetic acid (80 per cent)

This is applied to the wart which is covered with 40 per cent salicylic plaster, cut to the size of the wart. The patient is instructed to leave the dressing in place for at least 2–3 days and then remove it. The patient is seen again 7–14 days after application of the acid. It is then usually easy to 'shell out' most warts by curettage.

Treatment may be repeated if necessary. Delayed pain is a common complaint, and no more than three digits should be treated at the same time.

If the most aggressive destructive measures fail, or the patient is too squeamish, formalin may be applied daily with a wooden toothpick. If the lesions become inflammed, fissured, or tender because of the therapy or secondary infection, treatment is interrupted and a topical antiseptic used for several days.

Bleomycin

The effectiveness of intralesional bleomycin for recalcitrant warts is unquestionable. Bleomycin powder should be diluted to a final concentration of 1.0 U/ml with saline. Part of this solution will be further diluted to 0.1 U/ml according to the region and the recurrences.

There may be rare complications with the use of bleomycin. Transient or permanent nail dystrophy may appear if the nail matrix is infiltrated. Local Raynaud's phenomenon has been described in fingers and patients with vascular impairment should therefore not be treated. Prolonged local necrosis may occur. Patients should be warned that the bleomycin injection is painful.

Cantharidin

Cantharone Plus (30 per cent salicylic acid, 5 per cent podophyllin, 1 per cent cantharidin) is designed for topical application to the wart and a 1–3 mm margin around the wart by the physician in the office; occasionally the nail must be trimmed to expose subungual warts to the medication. When dry the wart is covered by a piece of Blenderm (a topical steroid in a transparent adhesive film). The resultant blister is painful and inflamed. The next day under local anaesthesia, the wart tissue is treated by curettage. This treatment is not recommended for use in young children due to difficulties in pain management.

Electrodesiccation

Electrodesiccation can produce unsightly scarring. Extirpation of subungual and periungual warts by blunt desiccation offers a surgical alternative when conventional measures fail.

Carbon dioxide laser

On fingers the warts must be followed down fully into the sulcus of the lateral nail fold. Using a minimally defocused beam of less than 1 mm spot size allows the complete tracing-out of the tumour. For subungual warts the laser should be used to ablate 'interfering' portions of nail plate and the wart can easily be vaporized subsequently. Complications such as permanent nail dystrophy after ablation of periungual warts are rarely observed.

Cosmetic treatment of nail dystrophies

The human nail, chemically similar to horn and hoof, is not essential for the survival of *Homo sapiens*, but it has many important functions that are crucial for the efficient use of the hands and feet. The nail is a prime source for the transmission of organisms, both macro- and microscopic, toxins, irritants and allergens. Maintaining nail cleanliness is essential to many aspects of health. The nail is also a focus of great importance; for many, cleanliness alone does not achieve aesthetic satisfaction. A multitude of products, implements and procedures are now on sale to enhance the appearance of nails (and, therefore, fingertips). While the cosmetic industry encourages and caters for the trappings of nail care and adornment, the motivation is probably innate; nail beautification was an established practice in societies long past; the long fingernail, often accentuated by gold and jewelled fingertip extenders, was indicative of high rank and station in society. Thus for social, cosmetic and cultural reasons and to aid normal function of digits with abnormal nails it is important to consider cosmetic and podiatric or chiropody treatment for dystrophies in which cure is not possible.

There are a great many nail conditions which need camouflage. Several factors should be taken into account:

- age of patient
- sex
- type and origin of the dystrophy
- affected part of the nail apparatus: nail plate or distal phalanx

Available cosmetic means used for disguising the nail dystrophies include:

- nail varnish; stick-on nail dressing
- preformed artificial nail
- sculptured artificial nail
- nail wrapping
- adaptable nail prosthesis
- abrader

Nail varnish

Nail varnish may hide any type of chromonychia in women (even very young) if the surface of the nail plate is smooth, or if it can be rendered so by fine sandpaper. The hue resulting from *Pseudomonas* nail infection is often hidden by nail varnish which may be kept on during the treatment with chlorox, and is a helpful therapy for this condition. Psoriasis may benefit from use of nail varnish in some aspects.

Stick-on nail dressing ('Press-on' nail polish)

This consists of a very thin coloured synthetic film with an adhesive which fixes it firmly to the nail. The changes produced on the nail vary considerably in intensity from patient to patient. Flaking, roughness, ridging, onycholysis, disappearance of the lunula, disorganization of the nail plate which is delaminated and broken off can be observed. Mild paronychial inflammation with loss of the cuticle may be seen.

In some instances 9 or 12 months will pass before the nails have entirely returned to normal. The effect on the nail is simply traumatic, not allergic—a combination of the impermeability of the adhering film and the cumulative trauma to the nail plate when the film is repeatedly pulled off.

Preformed artificial nails

Any dystrophy may be corrected by preformed artificial nails, providing that some natural nail plate surface is present to allow adequate adhesion. It is obvious that a severe dystrophy will prevent this and the usefulness of such a prosthetic nail is then limited. Local complications may appear when preformed artificial nails remain on for 3 or 4 days.

Distant allergic eczematous contact dermatitis may occur, more often due to the glue than to the prosthetic nail itself.

Sculptured artificial nails

Some natural nail keratin must be present for sculptured artificial nails to be used. It is first roughened with a burr; then the natural nail is painted with the acrylic resins hardening at room temperature and moulded on to it.

The prosthesis can be filed and manicured to shape. As the nail grows out, further applications of the self-curing acrylic resins can be made to maintain a regular contour.

Allergic contact dermatitis may appear, generally after 2–4 weeks of applications, as distant sensitization (face, eyelids) or local reactions (onychial and paronychial tissues). On patch testing, the patient may react strongly to the acrylic liquid monomer.

Nail wrapping

Essentially, the free edge of each nail is splinted with layers of a fibrous substance such as cotton wool, paper or plastic film and affixed with a variety of glues: after drying, the edge is fashioned to requirements and the nail is coated with enamel. The entire procedure is repeated every 2 weeks. Nail wrapping is useful but can do significant harm if the entire nail is covered because of the occlusive nature of the material used. Allergic reactions to cyanoacrylate nail preparations (painful paronychia, onychodystrophy, discoloration and even exceptional permanent nail loss) are rare, but may persist for more than a year.

Adaptable nail prosthesis

In a wide variety of cases ranging from deformed nails to complete loss of the distal phalanx, in women particularly, a silicone rubber thimble-shaped finger cover may be employed. The fixation is excellent. The device is easy to clean (plain soap), non-inflammable, and the formed nail takes varnish well.

Nail abrasion

Thick nails in diseases such as psoriasis, pityriasis rubra pilaris, and pachyonychia congenita can be abraded. Hyperkeratosis is prone to be associated with onychomycosis of the toes. Nail abrasion helps to expose the nail bed to antifungal chemicals, especially in the elderly where systemic treatment is not advisable. Abrasion is a good way to improve the contour of an abnormal nail, for example in onychogryphosis.

In selected cases of ingrowing toe nail, repeated thinning of the nail plate may be a useful conservative method in association with appropriate definitive treatment.

There are many products, implements and devices for maintaining clean, well-groomed nails to satisfy individual needs. These benefits are obtained with small risk. The physician can and should be well versed in nail care and adornment to aid patients in achieving an improved, positive self-image: when specific medical cure is shown to be impossible, he will then be in a good position to judge the value of cosmetic, chiropody or podiatry treatments.

Further reading

Psoriasis

Zaias N, Psoriasis of the nail unit. *Dermatol Clin* (1984) **2**:493–505.

Lichen planus

Scher RK, Lichen planus of the nail. *Dermatol Clin* (1985) **3**:385–99.

Onychomycosis

Davies RR, Everall JD and **Hamilton E,** Mycological and clinical evaluation of griseofulvin for chronic onychomycosis. *Br Med J* (1967) **iii**:464–8.

Hay RJ, Baran R, Moore MK et al, *Candida* onychomycosis—an evaluation of the role of *Candida* species in nail disease. *Br J Dermatol* (1988) **118**:47–58.

Hay RJ, Mackie RM and **Clayton YM,** Tioconazole nail solution—an open study of its efficacy in onychomycosis. *Clin Exp Dermatol* (1985) **10**:111–15.

Svjgaard, E, Oral ketoconazole as an alternative to griseofulvin in recalcitrant dermatophyte infections and onychomycosis. *Acta Dermato Vener* (Stockh) (1985) **65**:143–9.

Zaias N, Onychomycosis. *Dermatol Clin* (1985) **3**:445–60.

Index